Sleep Apnea in Children and Adults

Editors

STACEY L. ISHMAN
CAROL LI
REENA DHANDA PATIL

OTOLARYNGOLOGIC CLINICS OF NORTH AMERICA

www.oto.theclinics.com

Consulting Editor
SUJANA S. CHANDRASEKHAR

June 2024 • Volume 57 • Number 3

ELSEVIER

1600 John F. Kennedy Boulevard • Suite 1800 • Philadelphia, Pennsylvania, 19103-2899

http://www.oto.theclinics.com

OTOLARYNGOLOGIC CLINICS OF NORTH AMERICA Volume 57, Number 3
June 2024 ISSN 0030-6665, ISBN-13: 978-0-443-29406-8

Editor: Stacy Eastman
Developmental Editor: Malvika Shah

Otolaryngologic Clinics of North America (ISSN 0030-6665) is published bimonthly by Elsevier, Inc., 360 Park Avenue South, New York, NY 10010-1710. Months of issue are February, April, June, August, October, and December. Business and Editorial Offices: 1600 John F. Kennedy Blvd., Suite 1800, Philadelphia, PA 19103-2899. Customer Service Office: 6277 Sea Harbor Drive, Orlando, FL 32887-4800. Periodicals postage paid at New York, NY and additional mailing offices. Subscription prices are $478.00 per year (US individuals), $100.00 per year (US & Canadian student/resident), $623.00 per year (Canadian individuals), $679.00 per year (international individuals), $270.00 per year (international student/resident). For institutional access pricing please contact Customer Service via the contact information below. Foreign air speed delivery is included in all *Clinics*' subscription prices. All prices are subject to change without notice. **POSTMASTER:** Send address changes to *Otolaryngologic Clinics of North America*, Elsevier Health Sciences Division, Subscription Customer Service, 3251 Riverport Lane, Maryland Heights, MO 63043. **Telephone: 1-800-654-2452 (U.S. and Canada); 314-447-8871 (outside U.S. and Canada). Fax: 314-447-8029. E-mail: journalscustomerservice-usa@elsevier.com (for print support); journalsonlinesupport-usa@elsevier.com (for online support).**

Reprints. For copies of 100 or more of articles in this publication, please contact the Commercial Reprints Department, Elsevier Inc., 360 Park Avenue South, New York, NY 10010-1710. Tel.: 212-633-3874; Fax: 212-633-3820; E-mail: reprints@elsevier.com.

Otolaryngologic Clinics of North America is also published in Spanish by McGraw-Hill Interamericana Editores S.A., P.O. Box 5-237, 06500 Mexico D.F., Mexico.

Otolaryngologic Clinics of North America is covered in *MEDLINE/PubMed (Index Medicus), Current Contents/Clinical Medicine, Excerpta Medica, BIOSIS, Science Citation Index,* and *ISI/BIOMED.*

Contributors

CONSULTING EDITOR

SUJANA S. CHANDRASEKHAR, MD, FACS, FAAO-HNS, FAOS
Consulting Editor, Otolaryngologic Clinics of North America; President, American Otological Society; Past President, American Academy of Otolaryngology–Head and Neck Surgery; Partner, ENT and Allergy Associates, LLP; Clinical Professor, Department of Otolaryngology–Head and Neck Surgery, Zucker School of Medicine at Hofstra–Northwell, Hempstead, New York, USA; Clinical Associate Professor, Department of Otolaryngology–Head and Neck Surgery, Icahn School of Medicine at Mount Sinai, New York, New York, USA

EDITORS

STACEY L. ISHMAN, MD, MPH
Instructor, Division of Otolaryngology–Head and Neck Surgery, University of Wisconsin School of Medicine and Public Health, Madison, Wisconsin, USA

CAROL LI, MD
Assistant Professor, Division of Pediatric Otolaryngology, Department of Otolaryngology–Head and Neck Surgery, Cincinnati Children's Hospital Medical Center, University of Cincinnati College of Medicine, Cincinnati, Ohio, USA

REENA DHANDA PATIL, MD, MBA
Associate Professor, Department of Otolaryngology–Head and Neck Surgery, University of Cincinnati College of Medicine, Chief, Otolaryngology, Cincinnati VA Medical Center, Cincinnati, Ohio, USA

AUTHORS

CHRISTINA M. BALDASSARI, MD
Associate Professor, Department of Otolaryngology–Head and Neck Surgery, Eastern Virginia Medical School, Norfolk, Virginia, USA

SUHAS R. BHARADWAJ, MD
Resident, Department of Otolaryngology–Head and Neck Surgery, Eastern Virginia Medical School, Norfolk, Virginia, USA

JACQUELYN K. CALLANDER, MD
Resident Physician, Department of Otolaryngology–Head and Neck Surgery, University of California, San Francisco, California, USA

ROBSON CAPASSO, MD
Professor, Department of Otolaryngology, Head and Neck Surgery, Stanford University, Palo Alto, California, USA

JOLIE L. CHANG, MD
Associate Professor, Department of Otolaryngology–Head and Neck Surgery, University of California, San Francisco, California, USA

ALAN T. CHENG, BHB, MBChB, FRACS
Clinical Associate Professor, Discipline of Child and Adolescent Health, Faculty of Medicine, The University of Sydney, Sydney, New South Wales, Australia; Department of Ear Nose and Throat Surgery, The Children's Hospital at Westmead, Westmead, New South Wales, Australia

DOUG CHIEFFE, MD
Otolaryngology–Head and Neck Surgery, Massachusetts Eye and Ear Infirmary, Boston, Massachusetts, USA

MEGAN L. DURR, MD
Associate Professor, Department of Otolaryngology–Head and Neck Surgery, University of California, San Francisco, San Francisco, California, USA

TAYLOR S. ERICKSON, MD
Resident Physician, Department of Otolaryngology–Head and Neck Surgery, University of California, San Francisco, San Francisco, California, USA

JAMES D. EVERY, MD, BMedSci
Registrar in Otolaryngology Head and Neck Surgery, Department of Otolaryngology, Head and Neck Surgery, The Wollongong Hospital, School of Medicine, University of Wollongong, Wollongong, New South Wales, Australia

BEATRICE C. GO, MD
Resident, Department of Otorhinolaryngology, University of Pennsylvania, Philadelphia, Pennsylvania, USA

CHRISTOPHER HARTNICK, MD, MS
Benjamin Harry Peikin Chair, Otolaryngology–Head and Neck Surgery, Massachusetts Eye and Ear Infirmary, Director, Division of Pediatric Otolaryngology, Director, Pediatric Airway, Voice, and Swallowing Center, Professor, Harvard Medical School, Boston, Massachusetts, USA

JAVIER J.M. HOWARD, MD, MPH
Resident Physician, Department of Otolaryngology, Head and Neck Surgery, Stanford University, Palo Alto, California, USA

STACEY L. ISHMAN, MD, MPH
Instructor, Division of Otolaryngology–Head and Neck Surgery, University of Wisconsin School of Medicine and Public Health, Madison, Wisconsin, USA

SAMANTHA L. JAENSCH, MBBS
Clinical Associate Lecturer, Northern Clinical School, The University of Sydney, Sydney, New South Wales, Australia; Sydney Medical School – Northern, St Leonards, New South Wales, Australia

ERIC J. KEZIRIAN, MD, MPH
Professor-in-Residence, Department of Head and Neck Surgery, David Geffen School of Medicine at UCLA, Los Angeles, California, USA; Department of Head and Neck Surgery, Santa Monica, California, USA

ERIN M. KIRKHAM, MD, MPH
Assistant Professor, Department of Otolaryngology–Head and Neck Surgery, The University of Michigan, University of Michigan Medical Center, Ann Arbor, Michigan, USA

MIA KLASNER, FNP-BC, MSN
Family Nurse Practitioner, Department of Otolaryngology–Head and Neck Surgery, University of Miami Miller School of Medicine, University of Miami Health System, Miami, Florida, USA

DEREK J. LAM, MD, MPH
Associate Professor, Pediatric Otolaryngology Division, Department of Otolaryngology–Head and Neck Surgery, Oregon Health and Science University, Portland, Oregon, USA

NICHOLAS R. LENZE, MD, MPH
Resident Physician, Department of Otolaryngology–Head and Neck Surgery, The University of Michigan, University of Michigan Medical Center, Ann Arbor, Michigan, USA

CAROL LI, MD
Assistant Professor, Division of Pediatric Otolaryngology, Department of Otolaryngology–Head and Neck Surgery, Cincinnati Children's Hospital Medical Center, University of Cincinnati College of Medicine, Cincinnati, Ohio, USA

STUART G. MACKAY, MBBS, FRACS
Clinical Honorary Professor, Consultant Otolaryngology Head and Neck Surgeon, Department of Otolaryngology, Head and Neck Surgery, The Wollongong Hospital, School of Medicine, University of Wollongong, Illawarra ENT Head and Neck Clinic, Wollongong, New South Wales, Australia

MATTHEW MAKSIMOSKI, MD
Clinical Fellow, Division of Pediatric Otolaryngology, Cincinnati Children's Hospital Medical Center, Cincinnati, Ohio, USA

REENA DHANDA PATIL, MD, MBA
Associate Professor, Department of Otolaryngology–Head and Neck Surgery, University of Cincinnati College of Medicine, Chief, Otolaryngology, Cincinnati VA Medical Center, Cincinnati, Ohio, USA

MADELINE JACQUELINE LOUISE RAVESLOOT, MD, PhD, MSc
Medical Doctor, Department of Otorhinolaryngology–Head and Neck Surgery, OLVG, Amsterdam, the Netherlands

JILLIAN N. SANFORD, MD
Assistant Professor, Division of Pediatric Pulmonology and Sleep Medicine, Department of Pediatrics, Oregon Health and Science University, Portland, Oregon, USA

KATHLEEN M. SARBER, MD
Assistant Professor, Uniformed Services University of the Health Sciences, Bethesda, Maryland, USA; Chief of Sleep Surgery, Otolaryngology, Wilford Hall Ambulatory Surgery Center, San Antonio, Texas, USA

MARIA V. SUURNA, MD
Professor of Clinical Otolaryngology–Head and Neck Surgery, Department of Otolaryngology–Head and Neck Surgery, University of Miami Miller School of Medicine, University of Miami Health System, Miami, Florida, USA

ERICA R. THALER, MD
Professor and Vice Chair, Department of Otorhinolaryngology, University of Pennsylvania, Philadelphia, Pennsylvania, USA

SECKIN O. ULUALP, MD, MBA
Associate Professor, Department of Otolaryngology–Head and Neck Surgery, University of Texas Southwestern Medical Center, Director, Division of Pediatric Otolaryngology, Children's Health Dallas, Dallas, Texas, USA

KAREN A. WATERS, MBBS, FRACP, PhD, GCCM
Conjoint Professor, Discipline of Child and Adolescent Health, Faculty of Medicine, The University of Sydney, Sydney, New South Wales, Australia; Professor Karen Waters, SIDS and Sleep Apnoea Research, Respiratory Support Services, The Children's Hospital at Westmead, Westmead, New South Wales, Australia

Contents

Foreword: Nearly 200 Years of Sleep Apnea: We've Come a Long Way xiii

Sujana S. Chandrasekhar

Preface: Sleep Renewed: Innovations in Sleep Apnea Care for Adults and Children xv

Stacey L. Ishman, Carol Li, and Reena Dhanda Patil

Health Inequalities in the Diagnosis and Treatment of Obstructive Sleep Apnea in Children and Adults 353

Javier J.M. Howard, Robson Capasso, and Stacey L. Ishman

Our understanding of the prevalence of obstructive sleep apnea (OSA) in the United States is confounded by significant inequalities in diagnosis and treatment based on gender, race and socioeconomic status. Health literacy and cultural norms contribute to these inequities. Large gaps in data exist, as certain populations like Native Americans, Pacific Islanders, and sexual minorities have been sparsely studied, or not at all. Future research should aim to develop more inclusive diagnostic strategies to address OSA in diverse populations.

Home Sleep Testing versus Traditional Polysomnography: Pros and Cons 363

Beatrice C. Go and Erica R. Thaler

Obstructive sleep apnea (OSA) is associated with long-term cardiovascular and respiratory comorbidities and increased burden on the health-care system. Early and accurate diagnosis is essential to reduce physical and financial implications of the disease. Polysomnography uses neurophysiologic channels as well as basic respiratory and sleep parameters to best estimate the presence and/or severity of OSA. Although home sleep testing may have the potential for more variable results, it is a viable alternative to increase access to diagnosis of OSA and facilitate initiation of positive airway pressure.

Advanced Diagnostic Techniques in Obstructive Sleep Apnea 371

Seckin O. Ulualp and Eric J. Kezirian

Video content accompanies this article at http://www.oto.theclinics.com.

Optimal surgical and medical management of obstructive sleep apnea requires clinically reliable identification of patterns and sites of upper airway obstruction. A wide variety of modalities have been used to evaluate upper airway obstruction. Drug-induced sleep endoscopy (DISE) and cine MRI are increasingly used to identify upper airway obstruction sites, to characterize airway obstruction patterns, to determine optimum medical and surgical treatment, and to plan individualized surgical management. Here, we provide an overview of the applications of DISE and cine MRI in assessing upper airway obstruction in children and adults with obstructive sleep apnea.

Comorbid Insomnia and Sleep Apnea: Challenges and Treatments **385**

Kathleen M. Sarber and Reena Dhanda Patil

Insomnia and obstructive sleep apnea (OSA) are 2 of the most prevalent sleep disorders and frequently co-occur. Therapy can be challenging as treatment of 1 disease may worsen the other. Cognitive behavioral therapy for insomnia is the first-line treatment for insomnia and has been shown to improve compliance with positive airway pressure therapy. Other alternatives to OSA treatment may have higher acceptance in those with comorbid insomnia and sleep apnea (COMISA), such as mandibular advancement devices or emerging pharmacotherapies. Surgery, particularly hypoglossal nerve stimulation, appears to be well tolerated and may improve insomnia in those with COMISA. Otolaryngologists must be cognizant of the common presentation of COMISA in patients seeking surgical treatment and utilize a multidisciplinary approach to the treatment of these complex patients.

Management of Obstructive Sleep Apnea in the Infant and Newborn **395**

Jillian N. Sanford and Derek J. Lam

Obstructive sleep apnea in newborns and infants presents a unique challenge with distinct differences in sleep physiology, etiologies, and management compared to older children. The indications for and interpretation of polysomnography are less well defined in infants. There are also no broadly accepted clinical practice guidelines for treating sleep apnea in this age group. Etiologies include general causes of upper airway obstruction in infants such as laryngomalacia, micrognathia, and nasal obstruction in addition to adenotonsillar hypertrophy. Treatment strategies must be tailored to the specific anatomic features and comorbidities of the specific patients and often require a multidisciplinary approach.

Adenotonsillectomy for Obstructive Sleep Apnea in Children **407**

Samantha L. Jaensch, Alan T. Cheng, and Karen A. Waters

Obstructed breathing is the most common indication for tonsillectomy in children. Although tonsillectomy is performed frequently worldwide, the surgery is associated with a number of significant complications such as bleeding and respiratory failure. Complication risk depends on a number of complex factors, including indications for surgery, demographics, patient comorbidities, and variations in perioperative techniques. While polysomnography is currently accepted as the gold standard diagnostic tool for obstructive sleep apnea, studies evaluating outcomes following surgery suggest that more research is needed on the identification of more readily available and accurate tools for the diagnosis and follow-up of children with obstructed breathing.

Surgical Management of Pediatric Obstructive Sleep Apnea Beyond Adenotonsillectomy: The Nose, Nasopharynx, and Palate 421

Nicholas R. Lenze, Suhas R. Bharadwaj, Christina M. Baldassari, and Erin M. Kirkham

While adenotonsillectomy is the primary treatment of pediatric obstructive sleep apnea (OSA), persistent OSA after surgery is common and may be due to residual obstruction at the nose, nasopharynx, and/or palate. Comprehensive evaluation for persistent pediatric OSA ideally includes clinical examination (with or without awake nasal endosocpy) as well as drug-induced sleep endoscopy in order to accurately identify sources of residual obstruction. Depending on the site of obstruction, some of the surgical management options include submucous inferior turbinate resection, septoplasty, adenoidectomy, and expansion sphincter pharyngoplasty.

Surgical Management of Pediatric Obstructive Sleep Apnea Beyond Tonsillectomy & Adenoidectomy: Tongue Base and Larynx 431

Matthew Maksimoski and Carol Li

Pediatric patients with persistent obstructive sleep apnea (OSA) after adenotonsillectomy often have additional sites of upper airway obstruction such as the tongue base or larynx. Sleep endoscopy and cross-sectional, dynamic imaging can be used to direct surgical management of persistent OSA. The tongue base is one of the most common sites of obstruction in children with persistent OSA, especially for patients with Trisomy 21. Lingual tonsillectomy, tongue suspension, and/or posterior midline glossectomy may be used to address lingual tonsil hypertrophy and tongue base obstruction. Epiglottopexy and/or supraglottoplasty may be used to address laryngomalacia and epiglottic prolapse resulting in OSA.

Neurostimulation for Pediatric Obstructive Sleep Apnea 447

Doug Chieffe and Christopher Hartnick

Up to 80% of children with Down syndrome (DS) are affected by obstructive sleep apnea (OSA), and only 16% to 30% will have resolution of their OSA with adenotonsillectomy. Hypoglossal nerve stimulation is a well-established therapy for adults with OSA and was recently approved by the Food and Drug Administration for use in children with DS and residual OSA. There is robust experience with this therapy in adults that has led to well-established care pathways. However, given the challenges inherent to caring for a complex pediatric population, these pathways are not directly transferrable to children with DS.

Neurostimulation for Obstructive Sleep Apnea 457

Maria V. Suurna and Mia Klasner

Neurostimulation of hypoglossal nerve has emerged as an effective treatment option of obstructive sleep apnea (OSA). Since FDA approval in 2014, therapy has been widely used in select patients with moderate-to-severe OSA who do not benefit from positive airway pressure. Ongoing research and technological developments continue to advance the therapy to deliver personalized and efficient treatment to patients with OSA.

Sex Differences in Obstructive Sleep Apnea Including Pregnancy and Response to Treatment 467

Taylor S. Erickson and Megan L. Durr

This article highlights the sex differences in obstructive sleep apnea (OSA) and sheds light on the varying presentations, diagnostic challenges, as well as treatment responses observed in men and women. The disparities in prevalence, manifestations, and therapeutic outcomes underscore the need for a nuanced approach to OSA diagnosis and management that considers sex-specific factors. Furthermore, this article highlights the importance of recognizing and treating OSA during pregnancy, as it poses unique challenges and potential risks to both maternal and fetal health.

Positional Treatment of Obstructive Sleep Apnea 481

Madeline Jacqueline Louise Ravesloot

Positional sleep apnea (POSA), a distinctive subtype of obstructive sleep apnea, underscores the critical influence of a patient's sleeping position on the severity of their condition. In the management of POSA, compliance with positional therapy (PT) is paramount, as it wields a profound impact on the treatment's efficacy and the overall alleviation of the disease. The advent of new-generation PT devices offers a promising alternative to conventional methods like the tennis ball technique, boasting higher compliance rates and substantial disease alleviation.

Treatment of the Nose for Patients with Sleep Apnea 491

Jacquelyn K. Callander and Jolie L. Chang

Nasal obstruction is common in patients with obstructive sleep apnea (OSA) and may variably impact symptoms and severity of OSA. It is associated with decreased continuous positive airway pressure (CPAP) compliance, and both medical and surgical management of nasal obstruction have resulted in increased CPAP adherence. Treatment of OSA with comorbid rhinitis via topical nasal steroids demonstrates a beneficial impact on daytime sleepiness. Isolated nasal surgery has been shown to result in decreased daytime sleepiness and snoring, with minimal effect on OSA severity.

Advances in Pharyngeal Surgery Over the Past 10 Years: New Techniques and Technology 501

Stuart G. Mackay and James D. Every

This article is a review of advances in pharyngeal surgery over the past 10 years regarding literature, surgical technique, assessment, collaboration, and future direction in the management of adult and pediatric obstructive sleep apnea.

OTOLARYNGOLOGIC CLINICS OF NORTH AMERICA

FORTHCOMING ISSUES

August 2024
Dysphagia in Adults and Children
Mausumi Syamal and Eileen Raynor, *Editors*

October 2024
Artificial Intelligence in Otolaryngology
Anais Rameau and Matthew G. Crowson, *Editors*

December 2024
Odontogenic Sinusitis
John R. Craig and Alberto M. Saibene, *Editors*

RECENT ISSUES

April 2024
Allergy and Asthma in Otolaryngology
Sarah K. Wise and Daniel M. Beswick, *Editors*

February 2024
Thyroid and Parathyroid Disease
Amy Y. Chen and Michael C. Singer, *Editors*

December 2023
Otolaryngologic Trauma
Sydney C. Butts, *Editor*

SERIES OF RELATED INTEREST

Facial Plastic Surgery Clinics
Available at: https://www.facialplastic.theclinics.com/

Foreword

Nearly 200 Years of Sleep Apnea: We've Come a Long Way

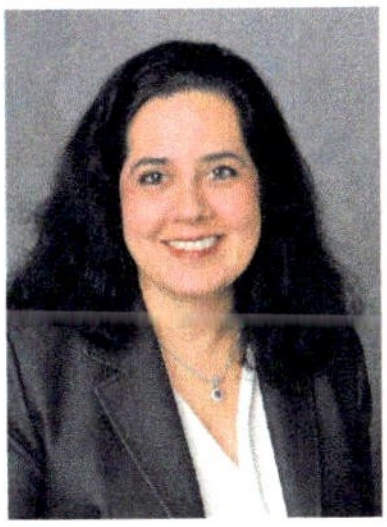

Sujana S. Chandrasekhar, MD, FAAO-HNS, FAOS, FACS
Consulting Editor

In 1836, the first installment of *The Posthumous Papers of the Pickwick Club* (also known as *The Pickwick Papers*), the first novel by English author Charles Dickens, was published. In it he introduces the reader to Joe, the Fat Boy, who is obese, consumes great amounts of food, constantly falls asleep in any situation at any time, is difficult to arouse, and snores. This description so intrigued the medical field that many hypotheses about the symptoms were examined, but it was not until well over a century after the novel was published that physicians started to interrelate these features. Joe's sleep problem is the origin of the medical term Pickwickian syndrome, which ultimately led to the subsequent description of obesity hypoventilation syndrome.[1]

Adult sleep apnea was first described in 1965 by Jung and Kuhlo.[2] Their description is that "the short diurnal periods of light sleep (10–12 seconds duration) in Pickwickian patients are characterized by apnea, increased cyanosis and muscular relaxation, simultaneous with sudden flattening of the EEG and slowing of the α-rhythm. The night sleep of Pickwickian patients is interrupted by long apneic periods of 20–40 seconds duration, terminated by 1–3 deep irregular snoring breaths." They go on to say that these patients rarely attain deep sleep stages, and long periods of rapid eye movements are lacking.

In 1892, Osler reported that children with "loud and snorting" respirations with "prolonged pauses" were often "stupid looking" and slow to respond to questions.[3] Nearly a century later, in 1976, Guilleminault and colleagues[4] performed polysomnography on eight children between ages 5 and 14, definitively describing pediatric sleep apnea.

Over the past several decades, understanding of central and obstructive sleep apnea in adults and children has progressed, with input from various disciplines, including otolaryngology, neurology, and pulmonary medicine. Likewise for developments of various treatments, surgical and nonsurgical alike. We also understand the systemic

Otolaryngol Clin N Am 57 (2024) xiii–xiv
https://doi.org/10.1016/j.otc.2024.02.026

ramifications of untreated sleep apnea. The worse the obstructive sleep apnea, the greater is the risk of coronary artery disease, heart attack, heart failure, and stroke. Obstructive sleep apnea also increases the risk of arrhythmias, which may lead to hypotensive events. Poor sleep is associated with a myriad of other issues that run the gamut of ill health.

This issue of *Otolaryngologic Clinics of North America* on Sleep Apnea in Children and Adults has been beautifully curated by the three co-Guest Editors, Drs Stacey L. Ishman, Carol Li, and Reena Dhanda Patil. The articles included emphasize compassionate, evidence-based, novel approaches to the diagnosis and treatment of sleep issues in all ages. The inclusion of discussions on social determinants of health care and special populations makes the issue particularly meaningful. I hope that you will find this a valuable resource.

Sujana S. Chandrasekhar, MD, FAAO-HNS, FAOS, FACS
Consulting Editor, Otolaryngologic Clinics of North America
President, American Otological Society
Past President, American Academy of Otolaryngology–Head and Neck Surgery
Partner, ENT & Allergy Associates, LLP

Clinical Professor, Department of Otolaryngology–Head and Neck Surgery
Zucker School of Medicine at Hofstra–Northwell

Clinical Associate Professor
Department of Otolaryngology–Head and Neck Surgery
Icahn School of Medicine at Mount Sinai
18 East 48th Street, 2nd Floor
New York, NY 10017, USA

E-mail address:
ssc@nyotology.com

REFERENCES

1. Kryger M. Charles Dickens: impact on medicine and society. J Clin Sleep Med 2012;8(3):333–8. https://doi.org/10.5664/jcsm.1930. PMID: 22701393; PMCID: PMC3365094.
2. Jung R, Kuhlo W. Neurophysiological studies of abnormal night sleep and the Pickwickian syndrome. Prog Brain Res 1965;18:140–59. https://doi.org/10.1016/s0079-6123(08)63590-6. PMID: 14329033.
3. Gozal D. Obstructive sleep apnea in children: implications for the developing central nervous system. Semin Pediatr Neurol 2008;15(2):100–6. https://doi.org/10.1016/j.spen.2008.03.006. PMID: 18555196; PMCID: PMC2490595.
4. Guilleminault C, Eldridge FL, Simmons FB, et al. Sleep apnea in eight children. Pediatrics 1976;58(1):23–30. PMID: 934781.

Preface

Sleep Renewed: Innovations in Sleep Apnea Care for Adults and Children

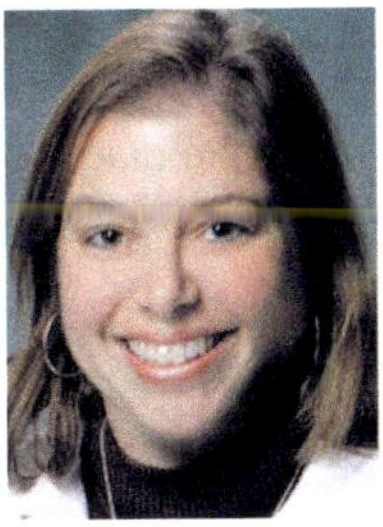
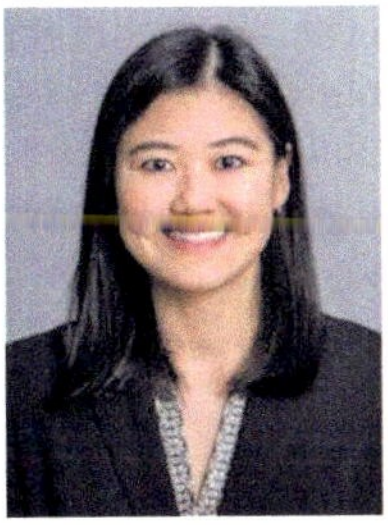
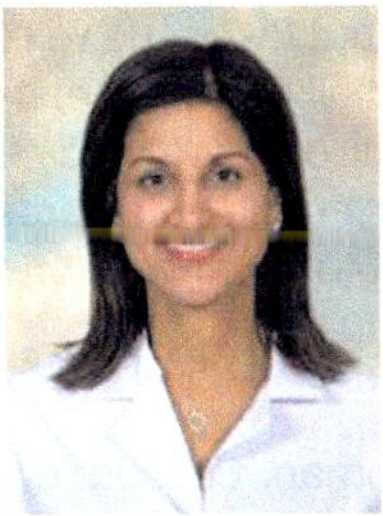

Stacey L. Ishman, MD, MPH   Carol Li, MD   Reena Dhanda Patil, MD, MBA
Editors

Welcome to our latest issue of *Otolaryngologic Clinics of North America* dedicated to advances in sleep disorders as they relate to surgical treatment in pediatric and adult populations. We offer this issue as a timely and relevant update regarding the treatment of sleep patients as our Otolaryngology community witnesses an increasing prevalence in sleep-disordered breathing. This affects millions worldwide, and it is evident that sleep disorders impact both individual health and societal well-being. Interestingly, this issue is the seventh *Otolaryngologic Clinics of North America* issue focusing on sleep disorders since the first one entitled "Sleep Apnea" published in August 1990 by Charles Koopmann Jr and Willard Moran Jr.

In this issue, we curated content evenly between pediatric and adult populations to highlight the latest research, the overlap in approaches between these groups, and interventions in patients of all ages. Our authors contributed a diverse array of articles over a wide spectrum of topics. We open the issue with an in-depth examination of how health inequalities and social determinants of health play into the diagnosis and treatment of obstructive sleep apnea (OSA). We emphasize the importance of patient selection for sleep surgery in OSA, particularly for patients with common sleep comorbidities such as insomnia. We then follow with five articles focused on children, starting with the management of OSA in newborns all the way to neurostimulation in the teen population—a procedure that was approved last year for children with Down syndrome. We then pivot to neurostimulation in adults, followed by articles focusing on sex differences in OSA (especially during pregnancy) as well as advances in positional therapy—which has advanced significantly from the days of sewing a tennis ball into a T-shirt to maintain side sleep. Finally, our authors have explored the latest in treatment

Otolaryngol Clin N Am 57 (2024) xv–xvi
https://doi.org/10.1016/j.otc.2024.02.018
0030-6665/24/Published by Elsevier Inc.

of nasal disorders and pharyngeal collapse to educate our readers on the pros and cons of various upper-airway surgeries.

In editing this issue, we aimed to provide a platform for our specialty's experts to share their insights based on their own research and practice. We are grateful for the dedication and expertise of our authors, editorial board members, and publishing team, whose collective efforts have made this journal a reality. In particular, we thank Dr Sujana Chandrasekhar for her leadership and guidance, as well our patient Editors and Staff at Elsevier Publishing, including Stacy Eastman and Malvika Shah. We extend our sincere appreciation to the broader Otolaryngology community for their ongoing support and commitment to advancing this important field.

We hope that this issue will serve as a valuable resource for clinicians, researchers, trainees, and all those interested in the intersection of sleep medicine and surgery. As a result of our ongoing study, let us continue to strive for excellence in the diagnosis and treatment of sleep disorders through evidence-based practice and innovation.

Thank you for joining us on this journey.

DISCLOSURE

Stacey L. Ishman: Ethicon, consulting; Carol Li: none; Reena Dhanda Patil: none.

Stacey L. Ishman, MD, MPH
Division of Otolaryngology–
Head and Neck Surgery
University of Wisconsin School
of Medicine and Public Health
K4/719 Clinical Science Center
600 Highland Avenue
Madison, WI 53792, USA

Carol Li, MD
Division of Pediatric Otolaryngology
Cincinnati Children's Hospital Medical Center
Department of Otolaryngology–
Head and Neck Surgery
University of Cincinnati College of Medicine
3333 Burnet Avenue
MLC 2018
Cincinnati, OH 45229, USA

Reena Dhanda Patil, MD, MBA
Department of Otolaryngology–
Head and Neck Surgery
University of Cincinnati College of Medicine
MSB 6507, 231 Albert Sabin Way
Cincinnati, OH 45267-0528, USA

E-mail addresses:
Staceyishman1@gmail.com (S.L. Ishman)
carol.li@cchmc.org (C. Li)
reenadhanda1@gmail.com (R. Dhanda Patil)

Health Inequalities in the Diagnosis and Treatment of Obstructive Sleep Apnea in Children and Adults

Javier J.M. Howard, MD, MPH[a,1], Robson Capasso, MD[a,1],
Stacey L. Ishman, MD, MPH[b,*]

KEYWORDS

- Obstructive sleep apnea • Inequalities • Disparities • Socioeconomic • Gender
- Race • Ethnicity

KEY POINTS

- The prevalence of obstructive sleep apnea (OSA) is increasing in the United States, with disadvantaged populations disproportionately affected.
- Biological sex influences OSA prevalence; estrogen may be protective, while testosterone may contribute to OSA development.
- There are significant disparities in OSA diagnosis and treatment based on gender, race, and socioeconomic status.
- Health literacy and cultural norms affect the recognition and management of OSA, contributing to inequities in care.
- Future research should address the gaps in understanding OSA in diverse populations and develop inclusive diagnostic strategies.

INTRODUCTION

In the United States, the prevalence of obstructive sleep apnea (OSA) is growing across the board in tandem with the obesity epidemic.[1,2] There is a growing body of evidence asserting that disadvantaged populations are disproportionately impacted by OSA, much like a myriad of other chronic diseases. We seek to characterize the English-language literature exploring the health inequities in the diagnosis and treatment of OSA across the lifespan.

Funding: This work was not funded.
[a] Department of Otolaryngology, Head and Neck Surgery, Stanford University, Palo Alto, CA, USA; [b] Division of Otolaryngology – Head and Neck Surgery, University of Wisconsin School of Medicine and Public Health, Madison, WI, USA
[1] Present address: 801 Welch Road, Palo Alto, CA 94304.
* Corresponding author. University of Wisconsin School of Medicine and Public Health, K4/719 Clinical Science Center, 600 Highland Avenue, Madison, WI 53792.
E-mail address: staceyishman1@gmail.com

Otolaryngol Clin N Am 57 (2024) 353–362
https://doi.org/10.1016/j.otc.2024.02.004
oto.theclinics.com

SEX

With regards to biological sex, the evidence to date illustrates that estrogen likely plays a protective role against OSA development.[1,3–5] Explanations from animal and in vitro studies demonstrate estrogen receptor up regulation in the genioglossus muscle, which they hypothesize may be protective on the fatigability of the muscle when exposed to intermittent hypoxia.[4] A handful of small human case series support this hypothesis along with larger scale population of data. An even smaller number of weak studies support the theory that testosterone may play a role in the pathogenesis of OSA.[6,7] Epidemiologic assessments report that men have a 2:1 or 3:1 predominance of OSA when matched with their premenopausal peers, but the relationship is 1:1 when they are compared to postmenopausal matches.[1,8,9] Of note, the prevalence and severity of OSA increases with age in both sexes.

In children, the data are quite limited. Because many studies rely on caregiver report of subjective sleep disordered breathing (SDB) symptoms for prevalence estimates, there is concern that these data are faulty with arguments for both over and underestimation. Similar to the data reported in adults, the symptom profiles of male and female children with OSA are influenced by social and cultural perceptions as to what constitutes normal age and sex-associated behaviors (snoring, hyperactivity, etc.). Additionally, the sample populations for these studies are often heterogenous, with unbalanced sex and age distributions that include both pre and postpubescent children. This last factor is considered critical as it has been widely theorized that differences in OSA prevalence between sexes likely emerge with puberty-related hormonal changes. The available evidence also suggests that boys have higher rates of SDB than girls, obese children have higher rates than those who are nonobese, and Black American children have higher prevalence rates than those who are not.[10]

Moreover, cultural norms and perceptions are also drivers of health inequities between men and women. The "classic presentation" of a patient with OSA was developed based on the presenting characteristics of middle-aged White men. Often, women presenting with OSA are described as having "more vague" symptoms than their male counterparts, including symptoms that overlap significantly with other common conditions like insomnia, hypothyroidism, and depression.[11–13] Of note, women with OSA are less likely to present with witnessed apneas (as hypopneas are more commonly prevalent in women) and typically report consuming less caffeine than men with OSA.[12] These factors may contribute to delayed diagnosis, misdiagnosis, or underdiagnosis of OSA in women. This is supported by the fact that women tend to be diagnosed with OSA at a later age, with more central obesity, and at a higher body mass index (BMI) than men; despite this, the AHI at the time of diagnosis is lower for women than men.[14,15]

Overall, evidence from the United States shows that women are less likely to be diagnosed with OSA than their male counterparts. This is in keeping with the Wisconsin cohort study estimates that approximately only 7% of women and 18% of men with at least moderate OSA hold a formal diagnosis.[16] Among those individuals found to have mild OSA on polysomnography, only 2% of women and 10% of men had a diagnosis.

With regards to the treatment of OSA, very little evidence exists illustrating differences by biological sex. While the rates of diagnosis of OSA clearly differ between the sexes, it is unclear whether there are any differences in the prescription of OSA treatment. The literature regarding continuous positive airway pressure (CPAP) compliance by sex is mixed with some studies showing higher, equal, and lower compliance rates in men than women, depending on the study.[17–22] There is no literature assessing differences in the prescription or compliance of oral appliance therapy by sex for OSA treatment.

Of the few studies that report the sex breakdown of patients who have undergone surgical management for OSA, the available evidence alludes to a vast disparity in surgical care delivered. A large, national database study examining individuals undergoing either soft tissue or skeletal surgery for OSA found that men were significantly more likely than women to undergo surgery.[23] Similarly, data regarding implantation of new technology like hypoglossal nerve stimulation therapy suggests that women are also being left behind at even higher rates, as men constitute the vast majority of individuals who have been implanted.[24–26] The only treatment that seems to favor access for women is based on a single large national database study that reported that patients undergoing jaw surgery for OSA are more likely to be women.[27]

GENDER IDENTITY AND EXPRESSION

There is currently no literature specifically reporting or examining the clinical presentation, diagnosis, or treatment of OSA in individuals who are gender nonbinary or nonconforming. There is, however, a recent administrative claims database study that reporting higher rates of all sleep disorders in gender nonconforming youth, and 3 times the odds of OSA in transgender youth as compared to their cisgender peers. Gender affirming therapy (GAT) is associated with reduced odds of other sleep disorders; however, there was no difference seen in the odds of OSA in transgender youth using GAT.[28]

SEXUAL ORIENTATION

Given that one of the common ways that people present with concern for OSA is based on bed partner concerns or brought up by the patient's bed partner during health care visits, the role of sexual orientation should not be overlooked. There is currently a paucity of information examining differences in the clinical presentation or diagnosis and management of patients who are sexual minorities. However, the 2019 next generation health study, a national longitudinal cohort study of US adolescents found that sexual minority female individuals reportedly significantly more self-reported daytime sleepiness and snoring than their heterosexual peers.[29] They also noted that these symptoms tended to be associated with overweight status and increased depressive symptoms, which suggests that the overall health status of sexual minority female individuals may be worse than in sexual majority female individuals.[29] There were no other studies identified by these authors that examined sleep health disparities among sexual minorities highlighting this an area that deserves further study.

RACE AND ETHNICITY

While race and ethnicity are frequently used in medical research, there is no formal agreement regarding their definitions that has resulted in confusion, misuse of the terms, and a lack of clarity regarding their use. Moreover, race is a social construct, without any biological basis, which has been historically defined primarily based on physical characteristics. Alternatively, ethnicity, while also considered a social construct, is typically defined as a set of cultural factors including ancestry, nationality, language, cuisine, and religion that specific communities share.[30] With regards to the definition and reporting of race and ethnicity in scientific literature broadly, there is an immense degree of inconsistency.[31] Unfortunately, the otolaryngology and sleep research to date are wrought with these same issues, as the majority of studies fail to report race or ethnicity at all.[32] For those studies that did report results based on race and ethnicity, the existing English-language literature on health inequities will be summarized here.

With regards to the prevalence of OSA based on race and ethnicity, most available data compare White and Black populations within the United States, with fewer examining Latinx and Asian populations. In addition, there is almost no data that include indigenous American populations or other American ethnic groups.

Most of the American literature demonstrates that Black Americans have a higher prevalence and severity of OSA than Whites across the lifespan.[33,34] However, this paradigm has been challenged recently, with growing evidence reflecting no significant difference in the prevalence or severity of OSA between adult Black and White populations.[35–38] Broadly, it is reported that Black Americans have significantly worse sleep quality and duration, as well as increased daytime sleepiness when compared to their White peers.[35] This asserts that a broader disparity in sleep health exists and warrants further study for a multidisciplinary approach to eliminating that disparity.

Studies looking at differences in diagnosis among children report that Black children's caregivers are more likely to present with concerns about OSA than White children's caregivers.[39] This may be the result of a variety of factors including environmental issues like poorer neighborhood air quality, or bed-sharing.

Black adults are reported to underreport all sleep problems including the use of sleep medicine, difficulty falling and/or staying asleep, early morning awakening or waking feeling tired, and napping.[40] Despite that, Black adults were noted to be younger and have a higher BMI than their White peers at the time of diagnosis.[41] There are mixed data whether or not Blacks have more severe OSA at the time of diagnosis.[41,42]

Studies reporting on OSA prevalence in Latinx adults date back to the early 1990s with several reports noting that Latinx adults having significantly higher rates of OSA diagnosis and worse disease severity of OSA than non-Hispanic white populations; however, a majority of the more recent cohort studies have not found a difference in OSA prevalence among Latinx adults.[36,38,43,44] One study did, however, report a higher prevalence of severe OSA (apnea hypopnea index [AHI] >30) in Latinx adults when compared to non-Hispanic White Americans after adjusting for age and gender.[35] Latinx women with OSA were more likely to present with concurrent psychogenic insomnia, while White women with OSA were more likely to present with sleep maintenance insomnia.[13]

Reports of prevalence in Latinx children are scant. A single 2004 study found that Latinx children presented with greater caregiver-reported snoring, excessive sleepiness, witnessed apneas, and parent-reported learning difficulties than their White peers.[45]

Assessment of Asian American adults reports that they have a higher prevalence and severity of OSA relative to White American populations.[46,47] This may, however, vary based on nationality or ethnicity. In one large cohort study, Chinese Americans were found to have a higher odds of OSA in every severity category than White Americans, but had significantly lower odds of having a formal diagnosis of OSA.[35] Chinese individuals also tend to have a more severe OSA phenotype at a lower BMI than White adults, which may be due to craniofacial skeletal restriction.[48,49] Japanese Americans, on the other hand, are reported to have a lower prevalence and reduced severity of OSA than White Americans.[35,50]

Overall, Asian American adults tend to underreport sleep problems.[47] There is scant existing evidence on the differences in OSA symptoms reported between Asian and White children's caregivers.[10,51]

Very little-or-no data have been published comparing OSA prevalence or diagnosis for indigenous Americans, Pacific Islanders, or other ethnicities within the United States.

BEHAVIORAL AND SOCIOCULTURAL

Limitations in health literacy play a significant role in the disparities in the diagnosis and management of OSA.[52] It is well known that patients and families with low health literacy face barriers all along the health care continuum: with greater difficulty locating providers and more challenges communicating with providers once they have successfully located one than families with high health literacy. Even informational brochures in the waiting room can miss the mark with more than 40% of low health literacy patients requiring assistance interpreting National Sleep Foundation and American Academy of Sleep Medicine brochures.[53] Often, standardized screening and diagnosis methods do not effectively identify patients with OSA, with some studies showing that more than half of adults reporting difficulty completing the Epworth Sleepiness Scale.[54]

SOCIOECONOMIC STATUS

Children with lower socioeconomic status (SES) are less likely to follow up with an otolaryngologist and ultimately to receive treatment for OSA.[51,55] For those children with lower SES who undergo treatment for OSA, they are more likely than their higher SES peers to have postoperative complications.[56]

In adults, those with higher SES have a higher likelihood of receiving treatment for OSA and are up to twice as likely to be compliant with CPAP therapy as their lower SES peers.[57–59] Patients of the highest income brackets are also most likely to undergo surgical treatment for OSA when compared to those in lower income brackets.[23]

ENVIRONMENT AND GEOGRAPHY

There are few publications regarding the impact of environmental factors, despite well-known importance of environment on health—most frequently and notably on lower SES populations.[60] Data from the National Health and Nutrition Examination Survey found a correlation between living in households with pets or mildew smell with having higher rates of self-reported OSA symptoms.[61]

Evidence supports that there can be delays in the diagnosis and management of OSA in both urban and rural children with OSA, for differing reasons. In rural populations, the physical distance from providers and facilities like sleep laboratories may play a key role. There is evidence that longer driving times are associated with lower odds of polysomnography (PSG) before surgical management of OSA in Canadian children.[62] Children residing in inner-city, urban settings are more likely to have public insurance—and experience significantly longer intervals from initial evaluation to PSG than those with private insurance; they are also reported to be twice as likely to be lost to follow up and to have delayed time to treatment of those with OSA.[63,64]

Infrastructural limitations can often be a rate-limiting step for patients who are connected to health care resources. It can take months to undergo formal polysomnography after referral, with longer wait times reported in underserved communities.[65] Research in urban Black adult populations suggests that home sleep testing could play a key role in reducing these barriers, but more research is needed to assess the impact on clinical outcomes.[66]

SUMMARY AND FUTURE DIRECTIONS

There are significant inequalities in the diagnosis and treatment of patients with OSA and research in this area is inadequate, thus limiting our ability to fully understand the health care needs and fixes that are required to address them. Characterizing where these inequalities exist and then further examining the reasons behind those inequalities requires thoughtful and meticulous efforts by researchers and clinicians. Shifting the paradigm toward improved inclusiveness and reporting requires engagement of stakeholders representing the various identities and backgrounds of those suffering from OSA in the development of newly tailored educational materials, screening tools, and diagnostic approaches.

In particular, there are glaring gaps in our understanding of OSA as it manifests in certain communities like indigenous Americans, Pacific Islanders, and sexual minorities. The accurate and consistent reporting of demographic data like sex, sexual orientation, race, ethnicity, and gender identity is critical for the identification of health disparities in all groups: as we cannot intervene on issues that we do not know exist. Further efforts to diversify the pipeline to academic medicine, and more specifically otolaryngology, are likely critical to alleviating these inequities—as the perspectives of individuals from underrepresented groups are paramount in efforts to bring the disparities seen in patients from their communities to light.

CLINICS CARE POINTS

- When evaluating and managing sleep apnea patients, individual patient factors must be taken into account even outside of anatomy and physiology including culture, environment, behavioral, and psychosocial factors
- It is important to acknowlege that historically, most of the research on obstructive sleep apnea diagnosis and management has been based on overwhelmingly white, male populations
- Targeted efforts to engage diverse communities into the sleep care continuum are needed

DISCLOSURE

There was no funding for this work. Dr S.L. Ishman has consulted for Ethicon and has grant funding from NIDCR and NHLBI from the NIH. Dr R. Capasso serves on the Scientific Advisory Board for Invicta Medical.

REFERENCES

1. Bixler EO, Vgontzas AN, Lin HM, et al. Prevalence of sleep-disordered breathing in women: effects of gender. Am J Respir Crit Care Med 2001;163(3 Pt 1):608–13.
2. Schwartz AR, Patil SP, Laffan AM, et al. Obesity and obstructive sleep apnea: pathogenic mechanisms and therapeutic approaches. Proc Am Thorac Soc 2008;5(2):185–92.
3. Pickett CK, Regensteiner JG, Woodard WD, et al. Progestin and estrogen reduce sleep-disordered breathing in postmenopausal women. J Appl Physiol Bethesda Md 1985 1989;66(4):1656–61.
4. Lu Y, Liu Y, Li Y. Comparison of natural estrogens and synthetic derivative on genioglossus function and estrogen receptors expression in rats with chronic intermittent hypoxia. J Steroid Biochem Mol Biol 2014;140:71–9.

5. Shahar E, Redline S, Young T, et al. Hormone replacement therapy and sleep-disordered breathing. Am J Respir Crit Care Med 2003;167(9):1186–92.
6. Hanafy HM. Testosterone therapy and obstructive sleep apnea: is there a real connection? J Sex Med 2007;4(5):1241–6.
7. Payne K, Lipshultz LI, Hotaling JM, et al. Obstructive Sleep Apnea and Testosterone Therapy. Sex Med Rev 2021;9(2):296–303.
8. Redline S, Kump K, Tishler PV, et al. Gender differences in sleep disordered breathing in a community-based sample. Am J Respir Crit Care Med 1994;149(3 Pt 1):722–6.
9. Young T, Shahar E, Nieto FJ, et al. Predictors of sleep-disordered breathing in community-dwelling adults: the Sleep Heart Health Study. Arch Intern Med 2002;162(8):893–900.
10. Lumeng JC, Chervin RD. Epidemiology of Pediatric Obstructive Sleep Apnea. Proc Am Thorac Soc 2008;5(2):242–52.
11. Eliasson AH, Kashani MD, Howard RS, et al, Integrative Cardiac Health Project Registry. Integrative Cardiac Health Project Registry. Fatigued on Venus, sleepy on Mars-gender and racial differences in symptoms of sleep apnea. Sleep Breath Schlaf Atm 2015;19(1):99–107.
12. Shepertycky MR, Banno K, Kryger MH. Differences between men and women in the clinical presentation of patients diagnosed with obstructive sleep apnea syndrome. Sleep 2005;28(3):309–14.
13. Subramanian S, Guntupalli B, Murugan T, et al. Gender and ethnic differences in prevalence of self-reported insomnia among patients with obstructive sleep apnea. Sleep Breath Schlaf Atm 2011;15(4):711–5.
14. Huang T, Lin BM, Redline S, et al. Type of Menopause, Age at Menopause, and Risk of Developing Obstructive Sleep Apnea in Postmenopausal Women. Am J Epidemiol 2018;187(7):1370–9.
15. Heinzer R, Vat S, Marques-Vidal P, et al. Prevalence of sleep-disordered breathing in the general population: the HypnoLaus study. Lancet Respir Med 2015;3(4):310–8.
16. Young T, Evans L, Finn L, et al. Estimation of the clinically diagnosed proportion of sleep apnea syndrome in middle-aged men and women. Sleep 1997;20(9):705–6.
17. Joo MJ, Herdegen JJ. Sleep apnea in an urban public hospital: assessment of severity and treatment adherence. J Clin Sleep Med JCSM 2007;3(3):285–8.
18. Pelletier-Fleury N, Rakotonanahary D, Fleury B. The age and other factors in the evaluation of compliance with nasal continuous positive airway pressure for obstructive sleep apnea syndrome. A Cox's proportional hazard analysis. Sleep Med 2001;2(3):225–32.
19. Woehrle H, Graml A, Weinreich G. Age- and gender-dependent adherence with continuous positive airway pressure therapy. Sleep Med 2011;12(10):1034–6.
20. Sin DD, Mayers I, Man GCW, et al. Long-term compliance rates to continuous positive airway pressure in obstructive sleep apnea: a population-based study. Chest 2002;121(2):430–5.
21. Gagnadoux F, Le Vaillant M, Goupil F, et al. Influence of marital status and employment status on long-term adherence with continuous positive airway pressure in sleep apnea patients. PLoS One 2011;6(8):e22503.
22. McArdle N, Devereux G, Heidarnejad H, et al. Long-term use of CPAP therapy for sleep apnea/hypopnea syndrome. Am J Respir Crit Care Med 1999;159(4 Pt 1):1108–14.

23. Ruthberg J, Summerville L, Cai Y, et al. Utilization of surgical treatment for sleep apnea: A study of health disparities. Am J Otolaryngol 2020;41(6):102670.
24. Khan M, Stone A, Soose RJ, et al. Does race-ethnicity affect upper airway stimulation adherence and treatment outcome of obstructive sleep apnea? J Clin Sleep Med 2022. https://doi.org/10.5664/jcsm.10068.
25. Strollo PJ, Soose RJ, Maurer JT, et al. Upper-airway stimulation for obstructive sleep apnea. N Engl J Med 2014;370(2):139–49.
26. Morse E, Dodhia S, Suurna M. Upper Airway Stimulation in Female Patients: Safety and Efficacy of a Novel Lateral Approach. Otolaryngol Head Neck Surg 2023;169(2):406–11.
27. Garg RK, Shan Y, Havlena JA, et al. Disparities in Utilization of Jaw Surgery for Treatment of Sleep Apnea: A Nationwide Analysis. Plast Reconstr Surg Glob Open 2016;4(12):e1047.
28. Gavidia R, Whitney DG, Hershner S, et al. Gender identity and transition: relationships with sleep disorders in US youth. J Clin Sleep Med JCSM 2022;18(11): 2553–9.
29. Luk JW, Sita KR, Lewin D, et al. Sexual Orientation and Sleep Behaviors in a National Sample of Adolescents Followed Into Young Adulthood. J Clin Sleep Med JCSM 2019;15(11):1635–43.
30. Lewis C, Cohen PR, Bahl D, et al. Race and Ethnic Categories: A Brief Review of Global Terms and Nomenclature. Cureus 2023;15(7):e41253.
31. Flanagin A, Frey T, Christiansen SL, et al. The Reporting of Race and Ethnicity in Medical and Science Journals: Comments Invited. JAMA 2021;325(11):1049.
32. Prakash Y, Ward LM, Jaleel Z, et al. The Use of Race and Socioeconomic Status Variables in Published Otolaryngologic Research. Ann Otol Rhinol Laryngol 2023; 132(7):721–30.
33. Ancoli-Israel S, Klauber MR, Stepnowsky C, et al. Sleep-disordered breathing in African-American elderly. Am J Respir Crit Care Med 1995;152(6 Pt 1):1946–9.
34. Redline S, Tishler PV, Hans MG, et al. Racial differences in sleep-disordered breathing in African-Americans and Caucasians. Am J Respir Crit Care Med 1997;155(1):186–92.
35. Chen X, Wang R, Zee P, et al. Racial/Ethnic Differences in Sleep Disturbances: The Multi-Ethnic Study of Atherosclerosis (MESA). Sleep 2015;38(6):877–88.
36. Song Y, Ancoli-Israel S, Lewis CE, et al. The association of race/ethnicity with objectively measured sleep characteristics in older men. Behav Sleep Med 2011;10(1):54–69.
37. Hall MH, Matthews KA, Kravitz HM, et al. Race and financial strain are independent correlates of sleep in midlife women: the SWAN sleep study. Sleep 2009; 32(1):73–82.
38. Baldwin CM, Ervin AM, Mays MZ, et al. Sleep disturbances, quality of life, and ethnicity: the Sleep Heart Health Study. J Clin Sleep Med JCSM 2010;6(2):176–83.
39. Rubens SL, Patrick KE, Williamson AA, et al. Individual and socio-demographic factors related to presenting problem and diagnostic impressions at a pediatric sleep clinic. Sleep Med 2016;25:67–72.
40. Jean-Louis G, Magai CM, Cohen CI, et al. Ethnic differences in self-reported sleep problems in older adults. Sleep 2001;24(8):926–33.
41. Scharf SM, Seiden L, DeMore J, et al. Racial differences in clinical presentation of patients with sleep-disordered breathing. Sleep Breath Schlaf Atm 2004;8(4): 173–83.

42. Thornton JD, Dudley KA, Saeed GJ, et al. Differences in Symptoms and Severity of Obstructive Sleep Apnea between Black and White Patients. Ann Am Thorac Soc 2022;19(2):272–8.
43. Kripke DF, Ancoli-Israel S, Klauber MR, et al. Prevalence of sleep-disordered breathing in ages 40-64 years: a population-based survey. Sleep 1997;20(1):65–76.
44. Yamagishi K, Ohira T, Nakano H, et al. Cross-cultural comparison of the sleep-disordered breathing prevalence among Americans and Japanese. Eur Respir J 2010;36(2):379–84.
45. Goodwin JL, Kaemingk KL, Fregosi RF, et al. Parasomnias and sleep disordered breathing in Caucasian and Hispanic children – the Tucson children's assessment of sleep apnea study. BMC Med 2004;2:14.
46. Leong WB, Arora T, Jenkinson D, et al. The prevalence and severity of obstructive sleep apnea in severe obesity: the impact of ethnicity. J Clin Sleep Med JCSM 2013;9(9):853–8.
47. Ong KC, Clerk AA. Comparison of the severity of sleep-disordered breathing in Asian and Caucasian patients seen at a sleep disorders center. Respir Med 1998;92(6):843–8.
48. Liu Y, Lowe AA, Zeng X, et al. Cephalometric comparisons between Chinese and Caucasian patients with obstructive sleep apnea. Am J Orthod Dentofac Orthop 2000;117(4):479–85.
49. Lee RWW, Vasudavan S, Hui DS, et al. Differences in craniofacial structures and obesity in Caucasian and Chinese patients with obstructive sleep apnea. Sleep 2010;33(8):1075–80.
50. Genta PR, Marcondes BF, Danzi NJ, et al. Ethnicity as a risk factor for obstructive sleep apnea: comparison of Japanese descendants and white males in São Paulo, Brazil. Braz J Med Biol Res Rev Bras Pesqui Medicas E Biol 2008;41(8):728–33.
51. Boss EF, Smith DF, Ishman SL. Racial/ethnic and socioeconomic disparities in the diagnosis and treatment of sleep-disordered breathing in children. Int J Pediatr Otorhinolaryngol 2011;75(3):299–307.
52. Li JJ, Appleton SL, Wittert GA, et al. The relationship between functional health literacy and obstructive sleep apnea and its related risk factors and comorbidities in a population cohort of men. Sleep 2014;37(3):571–8.
53. Chesson AL, Murphy PW, Arnold CL, et al. Presentation and reading level of sleep brochures: are they appropriate for sleep disorders patients? Sleep 1998;21(4):406–12.
54. Ghiassi R, Murphy K, Cummin AR, et al. Developing a pictorial Epworth Sleepiness Scale. Thorax 2011;66(2):97–100.
55. Yan F, Pearce JL, Ford ME, et al. Examining Associations Between Neighborhood-Level Social Vulnerability and Care for Children With Sleep-Disordered Breathing. Otolaryngol Head Neck Surg 2022;166(6):1118–26.
56. Bhattacharyya N, Shapiro NL. Associations between socioeconomic status and race with complications after tonsillectomy in children. Otolaryngol Head Neck Surg 2014;151(6):1055–60.
57. Platt AB, Field SH, Asch DA, et al. Neighborhood of residence is associated with daily adherence to CPAP therapy. Sleep 2009;32(6):799–806.
58. Billings ME, Auckley D, Benca R, et al. Race and residential socioeconomics as predictors of CPAP adherence. Sleep 2011;34(12):1653–8.

59. Simon-Tuval T, Reuveni H, Greenberg-Dotan S, et al. Low socioeconomic status is a risk factor for CPAP acceptance among adult OSAS patients requiring treatment. Sleep 2009;32(4):545–52.
60. Evans GW, Kantrowitz E. Socioeconomic status and health: the potential role of environmental risk exposure. Annu Rev Public Health 2002;23:303–31.
61. Ansarin K, Sahebi L, Sabur S. Obstructive sleep apnea syndrome: complaints and housing characteristics in a population in the United States. Sao Paulo Med J Rev Paul Med 2013;131(4):220–7.
62. Radhakrishnan D, Knight B, Gozdyra P, et al. Geographic disparities in performance of pediatric polysomnography to diagnose obstructive sleep apnea in a universal access health care system. Int J Pediatr Otorhinolaryngol 2021;147:110803.
63. Harris VC, Links AR, Kim JM, et al. Follow up and Time to Treatment in an Urban Cohort of Children with Sleep-disordered Breathing. Otolaryngol Head Neck Surg 2018;159(2):371–8.
64. Boss EF, Benke JR, Tunkel DE, et al. Public insurance and timing of polysomnography and surgical care for children with sleep-disordered breathing. JAMA Otolaryngol Head Neck Surg 2015;141(2):106–11.
65. Medicine I of Policy B on HS Research C on SM. Sleep disorders and sleep deprivation: an unmet public health problem. Washington, DC: National Academies Press; 2006.
66. Garg N, Rolle AJ, Lee TA, et al. Home-based diagnosis of obstructive sleep apnea in an urban population. J Clin Sleep Med JCSM 2014;10(8):879–85.

Home Sleep Testing versus Traditional Polysomnography: Pros and Cons

Beatrice C. Go, MD, Erica R. Thaler, MD*

KEYWORDS

• Polysomnography • Home sleep test • Sleep study • Sleep apnea

KEY POINTS

- Although polysomnography (PSG) is the gold standard of diagnostic evaluation for obstructive sleep apnea (OSA), home sleep testing (HST) can be a more accessible, cost-effective alternative.
- PSG is more appropriate for patients with high suspicion of nonobstructive sleep disordered breathing than HST.
- Clinical history and physical examination in conjunction with an evaluation of patient characteristics and preferences are imperative for selecting the best modality to diagnose OSA.

INTRODUCTION

Early and accurate diagnosis of obstructive sleep apnea (OSA) is crucial to allow for the initiation of treatment and long-term management of symptoms. As OSA is associated with cardiovascular and metabolic disease, it is important to identify and stratify patients in a timely fashion not only to prevent chronic sequelae but also to lower subsequent financial costs on the health-care system.[1] Symptoms of OSA are widely variable, ranging from snoring and gasping events to daytime somnolence, fatigue, and decreased energy. The sleep study as an objective metric, therefore, is a more reliable and concrete method to evaluate sleep quality and associated disorders.

HISTORY/BACKGROUND

The sleep study was invented in the 1970s when clinicians integrated electroencephalography (EEG) technology with cardiovascular and respiratory parameters to create the overnight polysomnogram (PSG).[2] The PSG is traditionally administered in a sleep laboratory under the guidance of specialized and experienced technicians. With the

Department of Otorhinolaryngology, University of Pennsylvania, 3400 Spruce Street, Philadelphia, PA 19104, USA
* Corresponding author.
E-mail address: Erica.Thaler@pennmedicine.upenn.edu

Otolaryngol Clin N Am 57 (2024) 363–369
https://doi.org/10.1016/j.otc.2023.11.003 oto.theclinics.com
0030-6665/24/

advent of digitalization, the PSG was expanded to include electromyography (EMG), electrooculogram (EOG), and electrocardiogram (ECG) data to help assist in sleep staging and detection of arrhythmias. With the addition of pulse oximetry, end-tidal capnography, airflow, respiratory effort, and body position sensing, this collection of data allows for a detailed interpretation of sleep quality.[3] Pulse oximetry and capnography can be used to capture desaturations and hypoventilation syndromes. Airflow, as measured through an oronasal sensor, allows for the differentiation of apneas from hypopneas. A thoracic or abdominal belt can measure respiratory effort, helping to discriminate obstructive events from central respiratory ones. A body position sensor is used to determine any positional contributions to sleep apnea. Additional channels, including expanded EEG, EMG, esophageal pressure, and nasal cannula monitoring, have also been described.[4] Video monitoring allows for recording of events, movement disorders, and real-time adjustment of channels.

DEFINITIONS

The apnea-hypopnea index (AHI), defined as the total number of apneas and hypopneas divided by total sleep time (TST) in hours, is the primary diagnostic indicator of OSA. An AHI score of 5 or greater in adults suggests the presence of OSA; symptoms can be further classified into mild (5≤ AHI <15), moderate (15≤ AHI <30), and severe (AHI ≥30). Apnea is defined as a cessation in airflow greater than 10 seconds.[5] There is greater variability in the hypopnea definition, as the American Academy of Sleep Medicine (AASM) defines hypopnea as a 30% or greater decrease in airflow associated with 3% or greater reduction in oxygen saturation in contrast to the Medicare and Medicaid definition of a 4% or greater reduction in saturation.[6] Other important information reported in the PSG includes the oxygen desaturation index, sleep latency, sleep efficiency, rapid-eye movement (REM) sleep, and hypnogram architecture. A constellation of these findings can help clinicians identify potential contributors to sleep apnea and guide subsequent management plans.

Sleep studies are currently defined as 4 different types. Type I is the traditional in-laboratory, monitored test. Type II is the same as Type I but unattended. Type III includes leads for respiratory effort, airflow, oximetry, and electrocardiogram (EKG) and is unattended. Type IV has only 2 leads, one for oximetry and one for airflow, and is also unattended. **Table 1** depicts each type and leads used in each method.

Most home sleep studies are Type III studies. Therefore, sleep time is neither recorded nor staged. Total recording time may be the denominator in determining respiratory event frequency, rather than TST, thereby falsely lowering the index. Sensitivity and specificity

Table 1
Type of sleep studies

	Type I	Type II	Type III	Type IV
Airflow	X	X	X	X
Oxygen saturation	X	X	X	X
Respiratory effort	X	X	X	
EKG	X	X	X	
EEG	X	X		
EOG	X	X		
EMG	X	X		
Attended	X			

of testing with type III devices have been shown to be 87% to 96% and 60% to 76%, respectively, for an AHI greater than 5. For an AHI greater than 30, the sensitivity is 50% to 97% and specificity is 90% to 93%.[7] Home sleep tests with Type III devices have also been shown to have a false-negative rate of 13% to 20%. This is particularly true of mild-to-moderate OSA, as reflected in the data above.[8] This potential for false negatives has led home sleep testing (HST) to be considered as either a screening tool for OSA or a tool to follow outcomes of therapeutic interventions.

The advantages and disadvantages and appropriate roles for HST and PSG are further discussed in the following section. Appropriate patient selection and understanding of the benefits/limitations to both types of studies can help clinicians expedite diagnosis and therefore commencement of care.

DISCUSSION

One of the greatest advantages that PSG confers is increased data availability, which allows clinicians to use the test in patients with a high suspicion of sleep disorders other than OSA. The addition of neurophysiologic channels including EEG also allows for interpretation of sleep data in accordance with different phases of the sleep cycle. There are multiple sleep stages that the normal human progresses through nightly, including stage W (wakefulness), stage N1 (non–rapid-eye movement [NREM] stage 1), stage N2 (NREM stage 2), stage N3 (NREM stage 3), and stage R (REM sleep). Parasomnias, narcolepsy, nocturnal seizures, and restless leg syndrome are all sleep-related disorders that may present similarly with nighttime awakenings, daytime somnolence, and more. In patients with any hallmark symptoms, it is important to distinguish whether there are any comorbid sleep disorders before selecting and initiating treatment of OSA. The hypnogram is an additional aspect of the PSG that serves as a visual representation of sleep, reporting stages of sleep as a function of time. By including this data, PSG can therefore help distinguish REM-based sleep disorders from isolated OSA, which HST currently cannot. It should be noted that many wearables are using alternative metrics to EEG to assess sleep stage with increasing reliability. This technology may ultimately be incorporated into home testing to allow more complete sleep assessment. Other data that are available through in-laboratory testing, including arm and leg EMG leads in conjunction with video monitoring, can support a clinical diagnosis of REM behavior disorder and restless leg syndrome.

Specific patient comorbidities with a higher likelihood of sleep disordered breathing other than OSA (ie, hypoventilation, central sleep apnea, or sleep-related hypoxia) are recommended to undergo PSG. Patients with significant cardiorespiratory comorbidities, neuromuscular weakness, chronic opioid use, and history of stroke are at particularly high risk for misdiagnosis if they undergo HST rather than PSG. A meta-analysis by Kapur and colleagues[9] for the AASM reported an overall low quality of evidence when assessing primary articles describing the use of PSG versus HST in patients with heart failure and chronic obstructive pulmonary disease. However, given the increased suspicion for non-OSA in this population, the benefit of conducting a PSG for earlier and more accurate diagnosis outweighs the risks of an inaccurate outcome from HST. Therefore, the AASM recommends that HST be used in patients who are medically uncomplicated and who present with a history and examination suggestive of moderate-to-severe OSA. This would include patients with daytime sleepiness, witnessed apnea, loud snoring, and hypertension. Patients with significant cardiopulmonary disease, respiratory muscle weakness, opiate use, and history of stroke should start with an in-laboratory study. However, patients who are not medically stable enough or have mobility issues with obtaining a PSG could potentially benefit from HST as a front-line diagnostic test.

Compared with HST, in-laboratory PSG can more accurately capture the presence and severity of OSA. By relying on TST elucidated from EEG data, the PSG can better estimate the true AHI because the HST relies on total recording time to calculate a similar value known as the respiratory event index (REI). Because the TST is the denominator used to calculate AHI, the REI can theoretically be decreased and underestimate the presence and/or severity of the disease.[10] TST may also be similarly impacted by insomnia, a comorbidity that is difficult to assess on HST and may cause inaccuracies in diagnosis. A meta-analysis from 2006 included 18 studies and reported 10% lower than average respiratory disturbance index when comparing portable sleep studies with PSG (odds radio, 0.90; 95% confidence interval, 0.87–0.92).[11] Another study more than a decade later compared PSG-measured and HST-measured AHI and found that the mean difference ranged from −14.8 to 10.6 events per hour, suggesting a wide range in diagnostic accuracy.[12] There were more than 20 different portable devices studied in this study, all of which had variable outcomes depending on number of channels, settings, and severity of individual disease.

Other disadvantages of HST include variability in parameter collection and lack of availability of trained personnel to oversee the test. PSGs are performed in specialized sleep laboratories under the observation of experienced technicians that can adjust sensors if needed for optimal capture. There may be wide inconsistencies between patients in using the equipment at home and furthermore, no ability to adjust the sensors for the most accurate collection. Dislodgment of the device during the night and poor-quality signals may lead to inaccurate data collection, requiring patients to undergo repeat studies at additional inconvenience and cost.

Although in-laboratory testing has been validated during many years of use, there have been concerns about certain features of such testing. Patients are often unwilling to sleep overnight in a laboratory, and if they proceed, they are uncomfortable with extensive monitoring attached to their bodies, thus decreasing sleep quality during the testing session. This undoubtedly affects the results of testing and may inaccurately depict the patient's true sleep disordered breathing. With the advent of widely available home testing, patient are now able to undergo a similar study to evaluate suspected OSA in the comfort of their own homes and during their regular nighttime routines. However, despite the intuitive advantage of sleeping in the comfort of one's own home, several studies have not shown a significant difference in patient satisfaction with HST compared with PSG.[13,14] One study assessing more than 2500 patient surveys collected from a national database found that patients who underwent in-laboratory PSG were more likely to be satisfied compared with their counterparts even after adjustment for potential confounders including health status, insurance, educational level, and other social characteristics.[15]

From an economic standpoint, there may be an advantage to using HSTs. Costs of attended studies have grown over time, and insurers are sometimes unwilling to cover these costs. Although there is tremendous variation in cost, an average in-laboratory study is approximately US$3000 but can range from US$1000 to US$10,000.[16] Home sleep apnea testing has been performed during several decades, and because monitoring devices have become more sophisticated, home testing is now increasingly used as a viable alternative diagnostic option for OSA. The cost of a home sleep study can be as low as US$150, a significantly lower burden to the patient and health-care system. One systematic review including 35 economic evaluation studies comparing the 2 diagnostic methodologies found that both type III and type VI tests were cost-effective compared with PSG. Several trials included in this review also found that

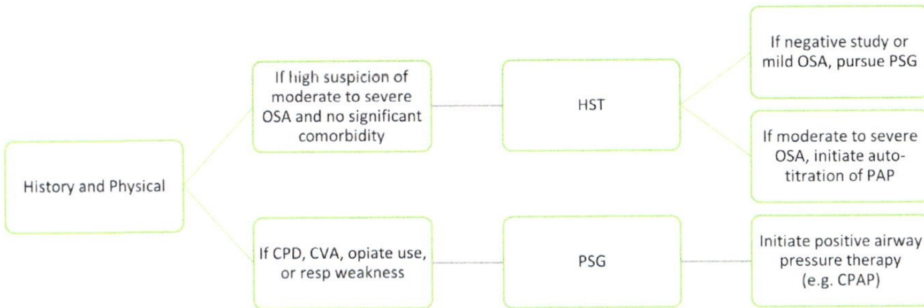

Fig. 1. Algorithm for sleep study ordering and utilization.

portable devices promoted access to care and reduced waiting times, thus potentially decreasing the indirect costs associated with late initiation of appropriate intervention of positive pressure.[17] Alternatively, the likelihood of underdiagnosis must be considered when using HST as the sole evaluator of OSA severity because there are also significant financial costs associated with repeat testing and false negatives. In highly populated, urban areas with decreased health-care resources, HST represents a potential solution to improve access to testing.

When comparing the efficacy of HST and PSG, a home-based strategy seems to be equivalent to in-laboratory PSG for autotitration of continuous positive airway pressure (CPAP). Before the advent of HST, after the diagnosis of OSA by an in-laboratory study, patients needed to attend another laboratory study for titration of appropriate pressure for treatment. One of the first studies comparing diagnosis and initiation of CPAP was a randomized controlled trial in 2007 comparing standard PSG with ambulatory CPAP titration in patients with high pretest probability of moderate-to-severe OSA.[18] After 3 months, there was no difference in AHI, Epworth Sleepiness Scale, and quality of life index but increased adherence to CPAP therapy was found in the ambulatory group. Similar findings were reported by the HomePAP study, which compared the use of HST versus PSG for autotitration of PAP to initiate CPAP prescription.[19] At 3 months, the HST group had significantly greater usage of CPAP by 1 hour and increased adherence to therapy by 12.6%. There was no difference in CPAP acceptance, fixed pressure, and number of effective titrations between both groups. Initiation of CPAP can be successfully titrated using a home-based strategy in adults with OSA without significant comorbidities, thereby lowering the need for laboratory-based titrations in this population (**Fig. 1**).

SUMMARY

PSG remains the gold standard for the diagnosis of sleep apnea due to its ability to diagnose alternate sleep disorders, to incorporate REM versus NREM data, and to accurately represent severity of OSA. In specific patient populations and clinical scenarios, PSG should be recommended over HST due to its reliability and standardization. However, as technology evolves with more accurate wearable measurements, HST may take on a more dominant role due to its increased availability, convenience, and decreased cost.

CLINICS CARE POINTS

- An accurate history and physical examination, as well as patient preferences, comorbidities, and clinical setting, are essential to the clinician when determining which diagnostic modality (PSG vs HST) for OSA is most suitable

- PSG should be used in patients with high suspicion of nonobstructive sleep disordered breathing conditions (ie, significant cardiorespiratory illness, neuromuscular weakness, chronic opioid use, and hypoventilation syndromes)
- The ability to calculate TST and close observation by experienced sleep technicians allows for increased diagnostic accuracy in PSG
- HST is a viable, cost-efficient diagnostic alternative in select patients with high suspicion for moderate-to-severe OSA without significant comorbidities
- In the appropriate patient, HST is a noninferior study that can be used to increase access to sleep testing
- Patients who have technically inadequate or nondiagnostic examinations on HST should undergo repeat testing with PSG

DISCLOSURE

There are no financial conflicts of interest to disclose.

REFERENCES

1. Kapur VK. Obstructive sleep apnea: diagnosis, epidemiology, and economics. Respir Care 2010;55(9):1155–67.
2.. Simons PJ, Overeem S. Polysomnography. In: Overeem S, Reading P, editors. Sleep disorders in neurology. Oxford, UK: John Wiley & Sons, Ltd; 2018. p. 13–29.
3. Rundo JV, Downey R. Polysomnography. Handb Clin Neurol 2019;160:381–92.
4. Markun LC, Sampat A. Clinician-focused overview and developments in polysomnography. Curr Sleep Med Rep 2020;6(4):309–21.
5. Park JG, Ramar K, Olson EJ. Updates on definition, consequences, and management of obstructive sleep apnea. Mayo Clin Proc 2011;86(6):549–55.
6. Berry RB, Abreu AR, Krishnan V, et al. A transition to the American Academy of Sleep Medicine-recommended hypopnea definition in adults: initiatives of the Hypopnea Scoring Rule Task Force. J Clin Sleep Med 2022;18(5):1419–25.
7. Jonas DE, Amick HR, Feltner C, et al. Screening for obstructive sleep apnea in adults: evidence report and systematic review for the us preventive services task force. JAMA 2017;317(4):415–33.
8. Rosenberg R, Hirshkowitz M, Rapoport DM, et al. The role of home sleep testing for evaluation of patients with excessive daytime sleepiness: focus on obstructive sleep apnea and narcolepsy. Sleep Med 2019;56:80–9.
9. Kapur VK, Auckley DH, Chowdhuri S, et al. Clinical practice guideline for diagnostic testing for adult obstructive sleep apnea: an american academy of sleep medicine clinical practice guideline. J Clin Sleep Med 2017;13(3): 479–504.
10. Light MP, Casimire TN, Chua C, et al. Addition of frontal EEG to adult home sleep apnea testing: does a more accurate determination of sleep time make a difference? Sleep Breath Schlaf Atm 2018;22(4):1179–88.
11. Ghegan MD, Angelos PC, Stonebraker AC, et al. Laboratory versus portable sleep studies: a meta-analysis. Laryngoscope 2006;116(6):859–64.
12. Abrahamyan L, Sahakyan Y, Chung S, et al. Diagnostic accuracy of level IV portable sleep monitors versus polysomnography for obstructive sleep apnea: a systematic review and meta-analysis. Sleep Breath Schlaf Atm 2018;22(3):593–611.

13. Berry RB, Hill G, Thompson L, et al. Portable monitoring and autotitration versus polysomnography for the diagnosis and treatment of sleep apnea. Sleep 2008; 31(10):1423–31.
14. Garg N, Rolle AJ, Lee TA, et al. Home-based diagnosis of obstructive sleep apnea in an urban population. J Clin Sleep Med 2014;10(8):879–85.
15. Kapur VK, Johnston JC, Rueschman M, et al. Patient satisfaction with sleep study experience: findings from the Sleep Apnea Patient-Centered Outcomes Network. Sleep 2018;41(8):zsy093.
16. Henry O, Brito A, Lloyd MC, et al. A Model for Sleep Apnea Management in Underserved Patient Populations. J Prim Care Community Health 2022;13. 21501319211068969.
17. Natsky AN, Chai-Coetzer CL, Vakulin A, et al. Economic evaluation of diagnostic sleep studies for obstructive sleep apnoea in the adult population: a systematic review. Sleep Med Rev 2022;62:101608.
18. Mulgrew AT, Fox N, Ayas NT, et al. Diagnosis and initial management of obstructive sleep apnea without polysomnography: a randomized validation study. Ann Intern Med 2007;146(3):157–66.
19. Rosen CL, Auckley D, Benca R, et al. A multisite randomized trial of portable sleep studies and positive airway pressure autotitration versus laboratory-based polysomnography for the diagnosis and treatment of obstructive sleep apnea: the homepap study. Sleep 2012;35(6):757–67.

Advanced Diagnostic Techniques in Obstructive Sleep Apnea

Seckin O. Ulualp, MD, MBA[a,b,*], Eric J. Kezirian, MD, MPH[c,d]

KEYWORDS

- Drug-induced sleep endoscopy • Cine MRI • Obstructive sleep apnea
- Airway obstruction • Children • Adults

KEY POINTS

- Drug-induced sleep endoscopy (DISE) and cine MRI are safe and useful techniques to assess levels of obstruction in children and adults with obstructive sleep apnea (OSA).
- Specific DISE findings are associated with outcomes of surgical treatment in adults.
- The utility of cine MRI in decision-making for OSA management in children and adults needs further exploration.

Video content accompanies this article at http://www.oto.theclinics.com.

INTRODUCTION

Obstructive sleep apnea (OSA) is characterized by repetitive episodes of upper airway obstruction leading to complete cessation or reduction of breathing, increased respiratory effort, altered gas exchange, and sleep disruption. Anatomic factors and upper airway motor tone result in upper airway obstruction due to dynamic airway movement and static obstruction.[1] Optimal surgical and medical management of OSA requires clinically reliable identification of patterns and sites of upper airway obstruction. A wide variety of modalities including, but not limited to, physical examination findings,[2–5] radiograph,[6–9] computed tomography,[10,11] MRI,[12] ultrasound,[13] flexible nasopharyngolaryngoscopy,[14,15] drug-induced sleep endoscopy (DISE),[16,17] and cine

[a] Department of Otolaryngology–Head and Neck Surgery, University of Texas Southwestern Medical Center, Dallas, TX, USA; [b] Division of Pediatric Otolaryngology, Children's Health, 2360 North Stemmons Freeway, F6.215, Dallas, TX 75207, USA; [c] Department of Head and Neck Surgery, David Geffen School of Medicine at UCLA, Los Angeles, CA, USA; [d] Department of Head and Neck Surgery, 1131 Wilshire Boulevard, Suite 302, Santa Monica, CA 90401, USA
* Corresponding author. Division of Pediatric Otolaryngology, Children's Health Dallas, 2360 North Stemmons Freeway, F6.215, Dallas, TX 75207.
E-mail address: seckin.ulualp@utsouthwestern.edu

Otolaryngol Clin N Am 57 (2024) 371–383
https://doi.org/10.1016/j.otc.2024.02.002
oto.theclinics.com

MRI[18–20] have been used to evaluate upper airway obstruction. To date, the gold standard method to assess upper airway obstruction in patients with OSA has not been established.

The complex and multifactorial nature of the pathogenesis of upper airway obstruction in OSA necessitates diagnostic tools reliably identifying the pattern, degree, and site of upper airway obstruction. DISE and cine MRI are increasingly used to identify sites of upper airway obstruction, characterize the patterns of airway obstruction, determine optimum medical and surgical treatment, and plan individualized surgical management. Here, we provide an overview of the applications of DISE and cine MRI in assessing upper airway obstruction in children and adults with OSA.

DRUG-INDUCED SLEEP ENDOSCOPY

The ideal diagnostic tool to evaluate upper airway obstruction in OSA would provide a real-time and dynamic assessment during natural sleep.[21] Since the feasibility of flexible fiberoptic endoscopy of the upper airway obstruction during natural sleep was reported in 1978,[14] few studies attempted to evaluate the mechanisms and patterns of airway obstruction during natural sleep.[22–24] Airway obstruction related to the palate, tongue, lateral pharyngeal wall, and epiglottis was documented during natural sleep.[14,22–24] Natural sleep endoscopy is impractical in daily practice and has limitations due to the wakefulness of patients during endoscopy and low depth of sleep when the scope was inserted in the nose.[24]

DISE overcomes the limitations of natural sleep endoscopy with the aid of sedation. DISE involves fiberoptic endoscopy of the upper airway during spontaneous breathing and sedation that attempts to share some similarities to natural sleep.[14,25] The upper airway obstruction patterns detected with DISE showed a moderate-to-good agreement with natural sleep endoscopy; however, the degree of obstruction during DISE was slightly higher than natural sleep endoscopy.[24] DISE is a safe and valid technique for identifying dynamic upper airway obstruction not seen on clinical examination.[26,27]

Indications of DISE in adults and children have been evolving, and they vary across different countries. In adults, indications for DISE may include the presence of OSA or snoring, positive airway pressure therapy failure, difficulty tolerating positive airway pressure therapy, and consideration of surgery, oral appliances, positional therapy, or combination approaches.[21,28] In children, indications for DISE may include the presence of OSA and small tonsils, persistent OSA after tonsillectomy and adenoidectomy, risk for persistent OSA after tonsillectomy and adenoidectomy, positive airway pressure therapy failure, difficulty tolerating positive airway pressure therapy, and additional sleep surgery planning.[29]

Technique

DISE is typically performed in the operating room with a comfortable room temperature, dimmed lights, and minimal noise disruption in adults and children with OSA.[21,30] Adults with OSA may have DISE in outpatient settings where personnel and appropriate equipment are available for the administration of sedation safely.[21] During DISE, patients should be monitored with a pulse oximeter, electrocardiogram, and blood pressure gauge. DISE can be performed in supine and/or lateral position depending on the clinical history.

The sedation level during DISE is critical to enhance the accuracy of DISE. Anesthetic agents alter the airway dynamics due to their dose-dependent effects on muscle tone, airway collapsibility, and airflow.[31] As anesthetic agents have a wide spectrum of action from sedation to general anesthesia, sedation depth influences the assessment of upper airway obstruction. While lighter sedation underestimates the upper airway obstruction, deeper sedation leads to artificial obstruction due to oversedation.[32–34]

A variety of anesthetic agents such as midazolam, propofol, dexmedetomidine, remifentanil, and ketamine, may be used to ensure optimal level of sedation during DISE, which refers to a state during which there is obstructive breathing and/or audible snoring and a lack of response to the stimulation of endoscopy. The effects of these agents on upper airway dynamics, nasal airway resistance, airway cross-sectional area, and respiratory drive vary.[35] The ideal choice of anesthetic agent achieving the targeted depth of sedation for DISE has not been identified. Given that no anesthetic produces natural sleep, we propose that sedation during DISE should produce upper airway physiology similar to natural sleep. In adults, propofol may achieve similar physiologic changes at the transition to unconsciousness.[36] In children, propofol and dexmedetomidine were identified as the optimal sedation agents in DISE, with the recommendation that inhalational agent use should be minimized.[29]

Interpretation

Obstruction at multiple levels of the upper airway can be assessed with the aid of DISE (**Figs. 1** and **2**). Several classification schemes and scoring systems are available to document, analyze, and report DISE findings in adults and children.[25,37–45] The majority of DISE scoring systems is developed for adults with OSA. In contrast to DISE classification systems for adults, DISE scoring systems for children include commonly known sites of obstruction in children with OSA, such as the nasopharynx and the larynx.[46] Assessment of the anatomic site, severity, and configuration of the obstruction varies among DISE scoring systems.[25,36–45]

The Velum, Oropharynx,Tongue base, Epiglottis (VOTE) classification is commonly used to report DISE findings in adults.[25] The VOTE system reports the degree (none, partial, or complete) and configuration (anteroposterior, lateral, or concentric) of the 4 anatomic structures most often contributing to pharyngeal airway obstruction: velum (ie, palate), oropharyngeal lateral walls, tongue, and epiglottis. The test–retest

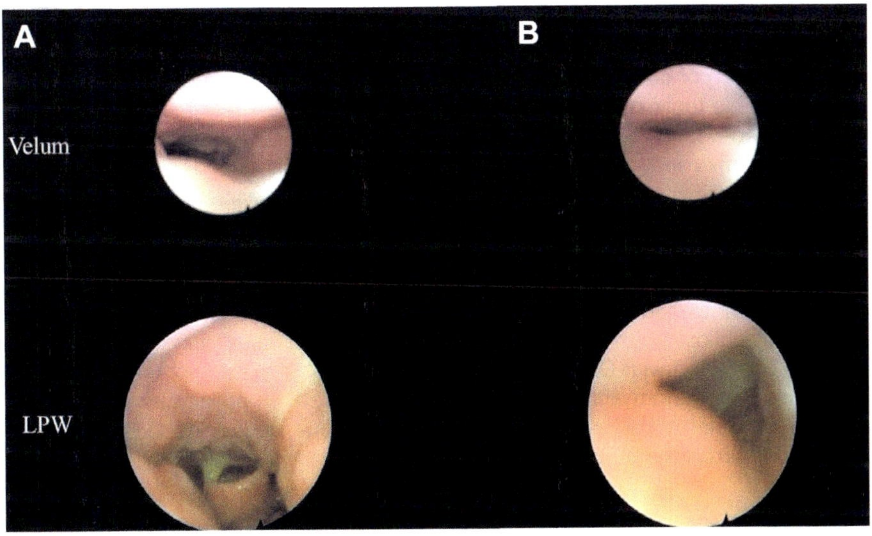

Fig. 1. Representative drug-induced sleep endoscopy images showing the open (*A*) and narrowed airway (*B*) at the levels of the velum and oropharynx/lateral pharyngeal wall (LPW).

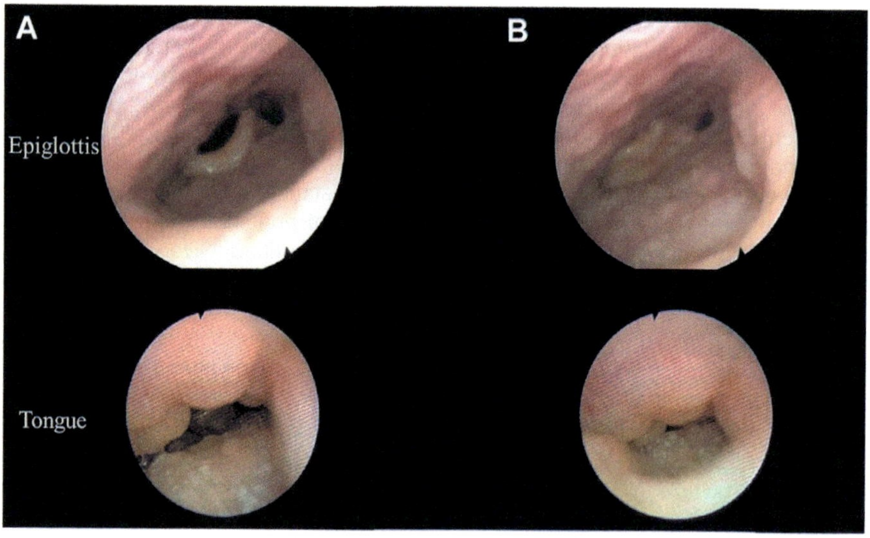

Fig. 2. Representative DISE images showing the open (*A*) and narrowed airway (*B*) at the levels of the epiglottis and tongue.

reliability of DISE is good with intraclass correlation coefficient analogs ranging from 0.41 to 0.89 for the palatal obstruction and from 0.57 to 0.84 for the hypopharyngeal obstruction.[47] The interrater reliability of DISE findings shows variation based on the degree and site of obstruction. The reliability of the detection of obstruction site is higher than for the degree of obstruction. The interrater reliability for the evaluation of the primary structure contributing to airway obstruction (0.70–0.86) is higher than for individual structures (0.42–0.71). The interrater reliability for the evaluation of the hypopharyngeal structures was higher than for those of the palate region.[48]

The interrater reliability of DISE assessment in adults varies between an experienced observer and a trainee, depending on the site of the obstruction.[49] The interrater agreement for the degree and configuration of the collapse is moderate to good for the majority of the sites of obstruction, and the agreement for the degree and configuration of collapse is good at the level of the tongue base. Nevertheless, DISE is a reliable technique even when assessing interobserver agreement between an experienced observer and a trainee.[49]

The comparative analysis of the DISE findings in children is limited due to dissimilarities among the DISE scoring systems used in previous studies.[50] DISE classification schemes and scoring systems in children included varying sites of upper airway obstruction and numerical scales. Furthermore, DISE technique and patient characteristics differed in the previous studies investigating DISE schemes and scoring systems in children.[50] Comparison of the DISE scoring systems in the same group of surgically naïve–healthy children with OSA revealed that none of the DISE scoring systems used in children correlated with OSA severity, age, and obesity.[51] Development of a practical DISE scoring system with good interrater and intrarater reliabilities while including all clinically pertinent anatomic sites contributing to upper airway obstruction has the potential to improve the utility of DISE in the management of children with OSA.

Clinical Applications

DISE in adults is used to identify the most appropriate alternative treatment option, reduce the rate of unnecessary surgical procedures, and improve treatment outcomes in adults with OSA who are unable to tolerate positive airway pressure.[21,51,52] In a few case series, DISE findings resulted in a change in surgical treatment plans in 40% to 78% of adults with OSA.[53–55] The use of DISE may reduce the rate of potential unnecessary surgery in adults with snoring.[55] Based on clinical examination, laser-assisted uvulopalatoplasty was recommended for 77% of adults with snoring; however, after DISE, laser-assisted uvulopalatoplasty was recommended for 54% of the patients who were a candidate for laser-assisted uvulopalatoplasty.[56] Similarly, DISE prevented potentially unnecessary treatment in 16% of adults with OSA.[53]

DISE is used to evaluate the site of airway obstruction in surgically naïve children and children with OSA after tonsillectomy and adenoidectomy.[57–60] In surgically naïve children, DISE provides information about the patterns of airway obstruction that can be used to counsel caregivers and plan surgical treatment.[57] Surgically naïve children with OSA may have single site and multiple sites of airway obstruction; the majority of children with OSA have obstruction at multiple sites of the upper airway. The most common sites of obstruction in children with OSA with multiple levels of airway obstruction are the combination of the oropharynx/lateral walls and velum obstruction. The most common site of obstruction in children with OSA with single-site airway obstruction is the oropharynx/lateral walls. Children with severe-or-moderate OSA exhibit complete obstruction at the velum and oropharynx/lateral walls more than children with mild OSA.[57] The effect of tonsillectomy and adenoidectomy on upper airway flow dynamics and sites of airway obstruction was documented in children with OSA who had DISE immediately after tonsillectomy and adenoidectomy.[58] Children with multiple sites of airway obstruction had residual obstruction in most of the sites; however, the degree of obstruction at the levels of the velum and oropharynx/lateral walls was significantly decreased after tonsillectomy and adenoidectomy.[57]

Children with Down syndrome have a similar rate of multisite obstruction compared with controls without obesity or Down syndrome.[59] However, children with Down syndrome demonstrate greater overall obstruction and greater tonsillar, tongue base, and arytenoid obstruction.[59] Children with obesity demonstrate less airway obstruction than those without.[58] Compared with nonobese children, obese children have similar airway obstruction at the velum, adenoid, lateral pharyngeal walls, tongue base, or supraglottis.[60]

Outcomes of Drug-Induced Sleep Endoscopy-Directed Therapy

The utility of DISE in targeted and effective treatment planning for OSA has been investigated in adults and children. In adults, DISE findings during the Esmarch maneuver correlate with the effect of mandibular advancement splint therapy and can be used as a prognostic indicator of successful oral appliance therapy.[61] While airway collapse at the base of the tongue during DISE has a higher rate of successful outcome for oral appliance therapy, the presence of complete concentric collapse at the velum or complete oropharyngeal lateral wall collapse has lower success rates with oral appliance therapy.[62]

Uvulopalatopharyngoplasty outcomes in patients with palate obstruction alone are better than in patients with hypopharyngeal collapse.[63–65] In a large, multicenter cohort study of adults undergoing sleep surgery, oropharyngeal lateral wall collapse and complete obstruction due to tongue were associated with poorer outcomes; however, tongue resection surgery seemed to improve outcomes in patients with complete tongue-related obstruction.[66] Multiple studies have shown that simply performing DISE does not guarantee successful outcomes; it is essential that we understand how to use DISE findings to select surgical procedures (and sometimes not to perform surgery at all).

In children, outcomes of DISE-directed surgical management of OSA have not been widely studied. Children with residual OSA after tonsillectomy and adenoidectomy (T&A) had subjective and objective improvement in sleep parameters after undergoing lingual tonsillectomy, midline posterior glossectomy, revision adenoidectomy, inferior turbinate submucosal resection, uvulopalatoplasty, or supraglottoplasty based on DISE findings.[67–70] In surgically naïve children with risk factors for residual OSA, DISE resulted in an intervention other than adenotonsillectomy (AT) in 58% of the children; DISE-directed surgical management achieved significant improvement in OSA.[71] In surgically naïve children with lateral pharyngeal wall collapse during DISE, the combination of modified expansion sphincter pharyngoplasty and adenotonsillectomy resulted in better outcomes than adenotonsillectomy in children with severe OSA.[72]

DISE findings are used to aid decision-making in hypoglossal nerve stimulation in children with Down syndrome and adults.[73,74] The primary role of DISE has been to exclude individuals with complete concentric collapse related to the velum, although the decision to adopt this approach was based on limited scientific evidence.[75] In a recent large, multicenter cohort study of adults undergoing treatment with hypoglossal nerve stimulation, complete tongue-related obstruction was associated with a greater odds of response, while complete (vs partial/none) oropharyngeal lateral wall-related obstruction was associated with lower odds of response.[76]

CINE MRI

Since the feasibility of cine MRI in evaluating the oral cavity and pharyngeal airway during sleep was reported in 1993, cine MRI has been increasingly used to evaluate airway obstruction in adults and children with OSA.[77] Cine MRI is also known as video MRI, FLASH MRI, ultrafast MRI, and dynamic MRI.[78] Cine MRI provides the assessment of the anatomy and dynamic airway motion without exposing individuals to ionizing radiation.

Technique

While cine MRI is commonly performed during natural sleep or drug-induced sleep in adults, cine MRI is conducted during drug-induced sleep in children with OSA.[78] In adults, natural sleep MRI is performed either late at night or after a period of sleep deprivation. Cine MRI in children is obtained after inducing sleep with propofol or dexmedetomidine.

Natural sleep MRI was accomplished with 65.93% of adults after a sleep deprivation period prior to attempting imaging. A variety of agents including, but not limited to, sedatives ranging from zolpidem, hydroxyzine, midazolam, chloral hydrate, or propofol are used to achieve sleep state for cine MRI in adults.[78]

Images are acquired while the patient is in a supine position with the cervical spine in the neutral position. The airway was imaged in the midline sagittal location from the nasopharynx to the level of the lower cervical trachea and in the axial plane at the level of the base of the tongue. Ultrafast images are displayed in a cine format to evaluate airway motion and obstruction (**Fig. 3**, Video 1).

Clinical Applications

Cine MRI in adults with OSA is used to evaluate airway obstruction patterns.[79–85] Different terminologies are used in describing the sites and degree of the obstruction. Sites of airway obstruction are reported as velopharyngeal, soft palate, retropalatal, retrolingual, retroglossal, hypopharynx, epiglottic, epipharynx, mesopharynx, and

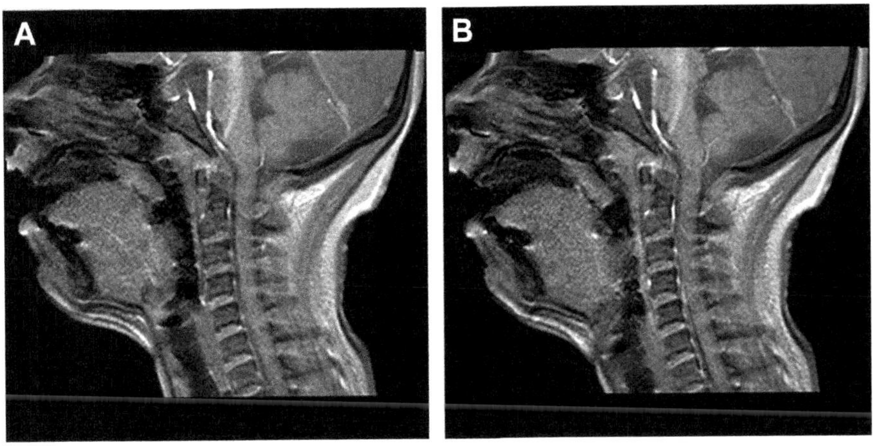

Fig. 3. Cine MRI showing upper airway obstruction. Sagittal images demonstrate the open (*A*) and narrowed airway (*B*) at the level of the tongue base (see Video 1). Cine MRI showing the posterior displacement of the tongue.

tongue base. Obstruction is reported as partial, complete, or deemed present when there 50% or 75% reduction in the length of the airway region. The common sites of airway obstruction in adults are retropalatal (98%), retroglossal (41%), and hypopharyngeal (5%) regions.[78] Lateral pharyngeal wall collapse is seen in 48% of adults with OSA. Multilevel obstruction involves the combination of retropalatal and retroglossal regions in 23.8% of adults with OSA and the combination of retropalatal, retroglossal, and lateral pharyngeal wall regions in 34.2%.[78]

Since the feasibility of cine MRI in children was reported in 2004, cine MRI has been used to evaluate airway obstruction in children with residual OSA after tonsillectomy and adenoidectomy.[18–20,86,87] The hypopharynx, tongue base, lingual tonsil, and macroglossia are the common sites of obstruction as detected with cine MRI.[20,87] In children with Down syndrome, adenoid regrowth and lingual tonsil hypertrophy are common causes of persistent upper airway obstruction documented during cine MRI.[19]

Compared with DISE, cine MRI shows the same upper airway obstruction site in the majority of children; however, DISE shows additional upper airway obstruction sites undetected by cine MRI.[20,87] Furthermore, nasal and supraglottic obstruction assessment is better with DISE as DISE is sensitive to partial versus complete collapse. Cine MRI provides a better overall view of primary and secondary airway obstruction while demonstrating soft tissue resolution for lymphoid tissue hypertrophy.[87] Nonetheless, cine MRI and DISE provide complementary information on the assessment of airway obstruction in children with residual OSA after tonsillectomy and adenoidectomy.[20,87]

SUMMARY

The complex and multifactorial nature of the pathogenesis of upper airway obstruction in OSA necessitates diagnostic tools reliably identifying the pattern, degree, and site of upper airway obstruction. DISE and cine MRI are increasingly used to identify upper airway obstruction sites, characterize airway obstruction patterns, determine optimum medical and surgical treatment, and plan individualized surgical management. Universally accepted indications, sedation protocols, classification schemes, and scoring systems are needed to optimize the role of DISE and cine MRI in clinical decision-making and counseling.

CLINICS CARE POINTS

- DISE and cine MRI are safe and useful techniques to assess levels of upper airway obstruction in children and adults with OSA.
- Specific DISE findings are associated with outcomes of surgical treatment in adults.
- Cine MRI and DISE provide complementary information on the assessment of airway obstruction in children with residual OSA after tonsillectomy and adenoidectomy.

DISCLOSURE

S.O. Ulualp has no conflicts of interest to disclose. E.J. Kezirian: Inspire Medical Systems—research funding; CryOSA: consultant, medical advisory board; Nyxoah SA: consultant; huMannity Medtec: consultant, Berendo Scientific: consultant, intellectual property; Magnap: intellectual property.

SUPPLEMENTARY DATA

Supplementary data related to this article can be found online at https://doi.org/10.1016/j.otc.2024.02.002.

REFERENCES

1. Ulualp SO. Snoring and obstructive sleep apnea. Clin North Am 2010;94:1047–55.
2. Davies RJ, Stradling JR. The relationship between neck circumference, radiographic pharyngeal anatomy, and the obstructive sleep apnoea syndrome. Eur Respir J 1990;3(5):509–14.
3. Stanford W, Galvin J, Rooholamini M. Effects of awake tidal breathing, swallowing, nasal breathing, oral breathing and the Muller and Valsalva maneuvers on the dimensions of the upper airway. Evaluation by ultrafast computerized tomography. Chest 1988;94(1):149–54.
4. Ingman T, Nieminen T, Hurmerinta K. Cephalometric comparison of pharyngeal changes in subjects with upper airway resistance syndrome or obstructive sleep apnoea in upright and supine positions. Eur J Orthod 2004;26(3):321–6.
5. Stauffer JL, Buick MK, Bixler EO, et al. Morphology of the uvula in obstructive sleep apnea. Am Rev Respir Dis 1989;140(3):724–8.
6. Sedaghat AR, Flax-Goldenberg RB, Gayler BW, et al. A case-control comparison of lingual tonsillar size in children with and without Down syndrome. Laryngoscope 2012;122(5):1165–9.
7. Gibson SE, Myer CM 3rd, Strife JL, et al. Sleep fluoroscopy for localization of upper airway obstruction in children. Ann Otol Rhinol Laryngol 1996;105(9):678–83.
8. Felman AH, Loughlin GM, Leftridge CA Jr, et al. Upper airway obstruction during sleep in children. AJR Am J Roentgenol 1979;133(2):213–6.
9. Fernbach SK, Brouillette RT, Riggs TW, et al. Radiologic evaluation of adenoids and tonsils in children with obstructive sleep apnea: plain films and fluoroscopy. Pediatr Radiol 1983;13(5):258–65.
10. Haponik EF, Smith PL, Bohlman ME, et al. Computerized tomography in obstructive sleep apnea. correlation of airway size with physiology during sleep and wakefulness. Am Rev Respir Dis 1983;127(2):221–6.

11. Guijarro-Martinez R, Swennen GR. Cone-beam computerized tomography imaging and analysis of the upper airway: a systematic review of the literature. Int J Oral Maxillofac Surg 2011;40(11):1227–37.
12. Nandalike K, Shifteh K, Sin S, et al. Adenotonsillectomy in obese children with obstructive sleep apnea syndrome: magnetic resonance imaging findings and considerations. Sleep 2013;36(6):841–7.
13. Isaiah A, Mezrich R, Wolf J. Ultrasonographic Detection of Airway Obstruction in a Model of Obstructive Sleep Apnea. Ultrasound Int Open 2017;3(1):E34–42.
14. Borowiecki B, Pollak CP, Weitzman ED, et al. Fibro-optic study of pharyngeal airway during sleep in patients with hypersomnia obstructive sleep-apnea syndrome. Laryngoscope 1978;88(8 Pt 1):1310–3.
15. Hori Y, Shizuku H, Kondo A, et al. Endoscopic evaluation of dynamic narrowing of the pharynx by the Bernouilli effect producing maneuver in patients with obstructive sleep apnea syndrome. Auris Nasus Larynx 2006;33(4):429–32.
16. Croft CB, Pringle M. Sleep nasendoscopy: a technique of assessment in snoring and obstructive sleep apnoea. Clin Otolaryngol Allied Sci 1991;16(5):504–9.
17. Kezirian EJ. Drug-induced sleep endoscopy. Operative techniques in otolaryngology–head and neck surgery 2006;17:230–2.
18. Donnelly LF, Shott SR, LaRose CR, et al. Causes of persistent obstructive sleep apnea despite previous tonsillectomy and adenoidectomy in children with Down syndrome as depicted on static and dynamic cine MRI. AJR Am J Roentgenol 2004;183(1):175–81.
19. Shott SR, Donnelly LF. Cine magnetic resonance imaging: evaluation of persistent airway obstruction after tonsil and adenoidectomy in children with down syndrome. Laryngoscope 2004;114(10):1724–9.
20. Clark C, Ulualp SO. Multimodality assessment of upper airway obstruction in children with persistent obstructive sleep apnea after adenotonsillectomy. Laryngoscope 2017;127(5):1224–30.
21. Charakorn N, Kezirian EJ. Drug-Induced Sleep Endoscopy. Otolaryngol Clin North Am 2016;49(6):1359–72.
22. Rojewski TE, Schuller DE, Clark RW, et al. Synchronous video recording of the pharyngeal airway and polysomnograph in patients with obstructive sleep apnea. Laryngoscope 1982;92(3):246–50.
23. Genta PR, Sands SA, Butler JP, et al. Airflow Shape Is Associated With the Pharyngeal Structure Causing OSA. Chest 2017;152(3):537–46.
24. Park D, Kim JS, Heo SJ. Obstruction Patterns During Drug-Induced Sleep Endoscopy vs Natural Sleep Endoscopy in Patients With Obstructive Sleep Apnea. JAMA Otolaryngol Head Neck Surg 2019;145(8):730–4.
25. Kezirian EJ, Hohenhorst W, de Vries N. Drug-induced sleep endoscopy: the VOTE classification. Eur Arch Oto-Rhino-Laryngol 2011;268(8):1233–6.
26. Lin AC, Koltai PJ. Sleep endoscopy in the evaluation of pediatric obstructive sleep apnea. Int J Pediatr 2012;2012:576719.
27. Berry S, Roblin G, Williams A, et al. Validity of sleep nasendoscopy in the investigation of sleep related breathing disorders. Laryngoscope 2005;115:538–40.
28. De Vito A, Carrasco Llatas M, Vanni A, et al. European position paper on drug-induced sedation endoscopy (DISE). Sleep Breath 2014;18(3):453–65.
29. Baldassari CM, Lam DJ, Ishman SL, et al. Expert Consensus Statement: Pediatric Drug-Induced Sleep Endoscopy. Otolaryngol Head Neck Surg 2021;165(4):578–91.

30. Bergeron M, Lee DR, DeMarcantonio MA, et al. Safety and cost of drug-induced sleep endoscopy outside the operating room. Laryngoscope 2020;130(8): 2076–80.
31. Chang JL, Goldberg AN, Alt JA, et al. International Consensus Statement on Obstructive Sleep Apnea. Int Forum Allergy Rhinol 2023;13(7):1061–482.
32. Heiser C, Fthenakis P, Hofauer B, et al. Drug-induced sleep endoscopy with target-controlled infusion using propofol and monitored depth of sedation to determine treatment strategies in obstructive sleep apnea. Sleep Breath 2017; 177:1006–744.
33. Maddison KJ, Walsh JH, Shepherd KL, et al. Comparison of Collapsibility of the Human Upper Airway During Anesthesia and During Sleep. Anesth Analg 2020; 130(4):1008–17.
34. Eastwood PR, Platt PR, Shepherd K, et al. Collapsibility of the Upper Airway at Different Concentrations of Propofol Anesthesia. Anesthesiology 2005;103:470–7.
35. Ehsan Z, Mahmoud M, Shott SR, et al. The effects of anesthesia and opioids on the upper airway: A systematic review. Laryngoscope 2016;126(1):270–84.
36. Hillman DR, Walsh JH, Maddison KJ, et al. Evolution of changes in upper airway collapsibility during slow induction of anesthesia with propofol. Anesthesiology 2009;111:63–71.
37. Pringle MB, Croft CB. A grading system for patients with obstructive sleep apnoea—based on sleep nasendoscopy. Clin Otolaryngol Allied Sci 1993;18: 480–4.
38. Camilleri AE, Ramamurthy L, Jones PH. Sleep nasendoscopy: what benefit to the management of snorers? J Laryngol Otol 1995;109:1163–5.
39. Vicini C, De Vito A, Benazzo M, et al. The nose oropharynx hypopharynx and larynx (NOHL) classification: a new system ofdiagnostic standardized examination for OSAHS patients. Eur Arch Oto-Rhino-Laryngol 2012;269:1297–300.
40. Bachar G, Nageris B, Feinmesser R, et al. Novel grading system for quantifying upper-airway obstruction on sleep endoscopy. Lung 2012;190:313–8.
41. Koo SK, Choi JW, Myung NS, et al. Analysis of obstruction site in obstructive sleep apnea syndrome patients by drug induced sleep endoscopy. Am J Otolaryngol 2013;34:626–30.
42. Boudewyns A, Verhulst S, Maris M, et al. Druginduced sedation endoscopy in pediatric obstructive sleep apnea syndrome. Sleep Med 2014;15:1526–31.
43. Chan DK, Liming BJ, Horn DK, et al. A new scoring system for upper airway pediatric sleep endoscopy. JAMA Otolaryngol Head Neck Surg 2014;140:595–602.
44. Lam DJ, Weaver EM, Macarthur CJ, et al. Assessment of pediatric obstructive sleep apnea using a drug-induced sleep endoscopy rating scale. Laryngoscope 2016;126:1492–8.
45. Qarbal J, Le Treut-Gay C, Allali L, et al. Drug-Induced sleep endoscopy in children: NAVOTEL scoring system development. Pediatr Pulmonol 2023;58(7): 1889–95.
46. Amos JM, Durr ML, Nardone HC, et al. Systematic review of drug-induced sleep endoscopy scoring systems. Otolaryngol Head Neck Surg 2018;158:240–8.
47. Rodriguez-Bruno K, Goldberg AN, McCulloch CE, et al. Test-retest reliability of drug-induced sleep endoscopy. Otolaryngol Head Neck Surg 2009;140(5): 646–51.
48. Kezirian EJ, White DP, Malhotra A, et al. Interrater reliability of drug-induced sleep endoscopy. Arch Otolaryngol Head Neck Surg 2010;136(4):393–7.
49. Carrasco-Llatas M, Zerpa-Zerpa V, Dalmau-Galofre J. Reliability of drug-induced sedation endoscopy: interobserver agreement. Sleep Breath 2017;21(1):173–9.

50. Tejan J, Medina M, Ulualp SO. Comparative assessment of drug-induced sleep endoscopy scoring systems in pediatric sleep apnea. Laryngoscope 2019; 129(9):2195–8.
51. Huntley C, Chou D, Doghramji K, et al. Preoperative drug induced sleep endoscopy improves the surgical approach to treatment of sleep apnea. Ann Otol Rhinol Laryngol 2017;126:478–82.
52. Stanley JJ. Drug-induced sleep endoscopy: techniques, interpretation and implications. Curr Opin Pulm Med 2020;26(6):623–8.
53. Eichler C, Sommer JU, Stuck BA, et al. Does drug-induced sleep endoscopy change the treatment concept of patients with snoring and obstructive sleep apnea? Sleep Breath 2013;17(1):63–8.
54. Gillespie MB, Reddy RP, White DR, et al. A trial of drug-induced sleep endoscopy in the surgical management of sleep-disordered breathing. Laryngoscope 2013; 123(1):277–82.
55. Fernández-Julián E, Garcia-Perez MA, Garcia-Callejo J, et al. Surgical planning after sleep versus awake techniques in patients with obstructive sleep apnea. Laryngoscope 2014;124(8):1970–4.
56. Hewitt R, Dasgupta A, Singh A, et al. Is sleep nasendoscopy a valuable adjunct to clinical examination in the evaluation of upper airway obstruction? Eur Arch Oto-Rhino-Laryngol 2009;266(5):691–7.
57. Ulualp SO, Szmuk P. Drug-induced sleep endoscopy for upper airway evaluation in children with obstructive sleep apnea. Laryngoscope 2013;123(1):292–7.
58. Mothersole K, Ulualp SO, Szmuk P, et al. The Effect of Tonsillectomy and Adenoidectomy on Upper Airway Obstruction Patterns in Children with Obstructive Sleep Apnea. Int Arch Otorhinolaryngol 2023;27(2):e211–7.
59. Hyzer JM, Milczuk HA, Macarthur CJ, et al. Drug-Induced Sleep Endoscopy Findings in Children With Obstructive Sleep Apnea With vs Without Obesity or Down Syndrome. JAMA otolaryngology– head & neck surgery 2021;147(2):175–81.
60. Lookabaugh S, McKenna M, Karelsky S, et al. Drug-induced sleep endoscopy findings in surgically-naïve obese vs non-obese children. Int J Pediatr Otorhinolaryngol 2020;138:110289.
61. Johal A, Battagel JM, Kotecha BT. Sleep nasendoscopy: a diagnostic tool for predicting treatment success with mandibular advancement splints in obstructive sleep apnoea. Eur J Orthod 2005;27:607–14.
62. Beeck S, Dieltjens M, Verbruggen A. Phenotypic labelling using drug-induced sleep endoscopy improves patient selection for mandibular advancement device outcome: a prospective study. J Clin Sleep Med 2019;15:1089–99.
63. Wang Y, Sun C, Cui X, et al. The role of drug-induced sleep endoscopy: predicting and guiding upper airway surgery for adult OSA patients. Sleep Breath 2018; 22:478–82.
64. Iwanaga K, Hasegawa K, Shibata N, et al. Endoscopic examination of obstructive sleep apnea syndrome patients during drug-induced sleep. Acta Otolaryngol Suppl 2003;(550):36–40.
65. Hessel NS, Vries N. Increase of the apnoea-hypopnoea index after uvulopalatopharyngoplasty: analysis of failure. Clin Otolaryngol Allied Sci 2004;29(6):682–5.
66. Green KK, Kent DT, D'Agostino MA, et al. Drug-Induced Sleep Endoscopy and Surgical Outcomes: A Multicenter Cohort Study. Laryngoscope 2019;129(3): 761–70.
67. Wootten CT, Chinnadurai S, Goudy SL. Beyond adenotonsillectomy: outcomes of sleep endoscopy-directed treatments in pediatric obstructive sleep apnea. Int J Pediatr Otorhinolaryngol 2014;78(7):1158–62.

68. Esteller E, Villatoro JC, Agüero A, et al. Outcome of drug-induced sleep endoscopy-directed surgery for persistent obstructive sleep apnea after adenotonsillar surgery. Int J Pediatr Otorhinolaryngol 2019;120:118–22.
69. Ulualp S. Outcomes of Tongue Base Reduction and Lingual Tonsillectomy for Residual Pediatric Obstructive Sleep Apnea after Adenotonsillectomy. Int Arch Otorhinolaryngol 2019;23(4):e415–21.
70. He S, Peddireddy NS, Smith DF, et al. Outcomes of Drug-Induced Sleep Endoscopy-Directed Surgery for Pediatric Obstructive Sleep Apnea. Otolaryngol Head Neck Surg 2018;158(3):559–65.
71. Kirkham E, Ma CC, Filipek N, et al. Polysomnography outcomes of sleep endoscopy-directed intervention in surgically naïve children at risk for persistent obstructive sleep apnea. Sleep Breath 2020;24(3):1143–50.
72. Ulualp SO. Modified expansion sphincter pharyngoplasty for treatment of children with obstructive sleep apnea. JAMA Otolaryngol Head Neck Surg 2014;140(9):817–22.
73. Strollo PJ, Soose RJ, Maurer JT, et al. Upper-airway stimulation for obstructive sleep apnea. N Engl J Med 2014;370:139–49.
74. Diercks GR, Wentland C, Keamy D, et al. Hypoglossal Nerve Stimulation in Adolescents With Down Syndrome and Obstructive Sleep Apnea. JAMA Otolaryngol Head Neck Surg 2018;144(1):37–42.
75. Van de Heyning PH, Badr MS, Baskin JZ, et al. Implanted upper airway stimulation device for obstructive sleep apnea. Laryngoscope 2012;122:1626–33.
76. Huyett P, Kent DT, D'Agostino MA, et al. Drug-Induced Sleep Endoscopy and Hypoglossal Nerve Stimulation Outcomes: A Multicenter Cohort Study. Laryngoscope 2021;131(7):1676–82.
77. Suto Y, Matsuo T, Kato T, et al. Evaluation of the pharyngeal airway in patients with sleep apnea: value of ultrafast MR imaging. AJR Am J Roentgenol 1993;160(2):311–4.
78. Volner K, Chao S, Camacho M. Dynamic sleep MRI in obstructive sleep apnea: a systematic review and meta-analysis. Eur Arch Oto-Rhino-Laryngol 2022;279:595–607.
79. Liu S, Huon L, Lo M, et al. Static craniofacial measurements and dynamic airway collapse patterns associated with severe obstructive sleep apnoea: a sleep MRI study. Clin Otolaryngol 2016;41:700–6.
80. Huon L, Liu SY, Shih TT, et al. Dynamic upper airway collapse observed from sleep MRI: BMI-matched severe and mild OSA patients. Eur Arch Oto-Rhino-Laryngol 2016;273:4021–6.
81. Moon IJ, Han DH, Kim J, et al. Sleep magnetic resonance imaging as a new diagnostic method in obstructive sleep apnea syndrome. Laryngoscope 2010;120:2546–54.
82. Chuang L-P, Chen N-H, Li H-Y, et al. Dynamic upper airway changes during sleep in patients with obstructive sleep apnea syndrome. Acta Otolaryngol 2009;129:1474–9.
83. Kavcic P, Koren A, Koritnik B, et al. Sleep magnetic resonance imaging with electroencephalogram in obstructive sleep apnea syndrome. Laryngoscope 2015;125:1485–90.
84. Moriwaki H, Inoue Y, Namba K, et al. Clinical significance of upper airway obstruction pattern during apneic episodes on ultrafast dynamic magnetic resonance imaging. Auris Nasus Larynx 2009;36:187–91.
85. Barrera JE, Chang RC, Popelka GR, et al. Reliability of airway obstruction analyses from Sleep MRI sequences. Otolaryngol Neck Surg 2010;142(4):526–30.

86. Schaaf WE Jr, Wootten CT, Donnelly LF, et al. Findings on MR sleep studies as biomarkers to predict outcome of genioglossus advancement in the treatment of obstructive sleep apnea in children and young adults. AJR Am J Roentgenol 2010;194:1204–9.
87. Li C, Kou YF, DeMarcantonio MA, et al. Sleep Endoscopy and Cine Magnetic Resonance Imaging Evaluation of Children With Persistent Obstructive Sleep Apnea. Otolaryngol Head Neck Surg 2023;168(4):848–55.

Comorbid Insomnia and Sleep Apnea

Challenges and Treatments

Kathleen M. Sarber, MD[a,b,*], Reena Dhanda Patil, MD[c,d]

KEYWORDS

- Obstructive sleep apnea • Insomnia
- Comorbid insomnia and obstructive sleep apnea (COMISA)
- Positive airway pressure (PAP) therapy • Hypoglossal nerve stimulation
- Cognitive behavioral therapy for insomnia (CBT-i) • Mandibular advancement device
- Sleep surgery

KEY POINTS

- Comorbid insomnia and sleep apnea (COMISA) presents commonly in patients seeking surgical treatment for obstructive sleep apnea (OSA).
- Insomnia and OSA share a bi-directional relationship and their co-occurrence synergistically worsens the effects of both disorders in COMISA, for example, adverse health outcomes and worsened mental health disorders.
- Treatment for patients with COMISA may be challenging due to issues with tolerance for and usage of OSA therapies (eg, positive airway pressure [PAP]).
- While COMISA is associated with lower rates of PAP tolerance, cognitive behavioral therapy for insomnia and pharmacotherapy have been shown to improve therapy compliance.
- Surgical treatment in COMISA may be a reasonable alternative to PAP therapy given elimination of the mask apparatus that can be disruptive to sleep and exacerbate insomnia.

INTRODUCTION

Insomnia and obstructive sleep apnea (OSA) are 2 highly prevalent sleep disorders and can co-occur in many patients.[1] Insomnia, according to the International

[a] Uniformed Services University of the Health Sciences, Bethesda, MD, USA; [b] Otolaryngology, Wilford Hall Ambulatory Surgery Center, 1100 Wilford Hall Loop, San Antonio, TX 78236, USA; [c] Department of Otolaryngology-Head and Neck Surgery, University of Cincinnati, 3113 Bellevue Avenue, Cincinnati, OH 45219, USA; [d] Department of Otolaryngology-Head and Neck Surgery, Cincinnati Veterans Affairs Medical Center, 3200 Vine Street, Cincinnati, OH 45220, USA

* Corresponding author. Wilford Hall Ambulatory Surgery Center, 1100 Wilford Hall Loop, San Antonio, TX 78236.
E-mail address: kathleen.m.sarber.mil@health.mil

Otolaryngol Clin N Am 57 (2024) 385–393
https://doi.org/10.1016/j.otc.2023.11.001
0030-6665/24/Published by Elsevier Inc.

Classification of Sleep Disorders third Edition (ICSD-3), is defined as a persistent difficulty with sleep initiation, duration, or consolidation that occurs despite adequate opportunity and circumstances for sleep and results in perceived daytime impairment such as fatigue, decreased mood or irritability, general malaise, or cognitive impairment.[2] Diagnostic criteria require that insomnia symptoms persist more than 3 days/week for a period of at least 3 months. The ICSD-3 defines OSA as greater than 5 predominantly obstructive respiratory events per hour of sleep in a patient with symptoms (daytime sleepiness, nonrestorative sleep, fatigue, waking with breath holding or gasping/choking) attributable to OSA or greater than 15 predominantly obstructive respiratory events with or without symptoms.[2] OSA results from a combination of anatomic factors that narrow the airway as well as non-anatomic factors such as a low arousal threshold, high loop gain due to hypersensitive respiratory control, and decreased airway muscle response to airway obstruction.[3] The contribution of each of these factors varies between individuals, and OSA phenotypes are a topic of much needed research.[3]

The presence of comorbid insomnia and sleep apnea (COMISA) was first reported by Guilleminaut in 1973 who documented 2 male patients with insomnia, severe sleep disturbances, and sleep apnea.[4] The reported prevalence of each disorder is approximately 6% to 10%,[5,6] making overlapping disease statistically less likely. However, studies show that COMISA is actually commonly encountered in clinical practice. In 1999, a study using polysomnogram (PSG) was performed on patients with insomnia to investigate the incidence of sleep disordered breathing. Of the 80 participants, 34 patients (43%) were found to have an apnea-hypopnea index (AHI) greater than 5.[7] Conversely, a 2001 study of patients who had undergone PSG and found to have clinically significant sleep disordered breathing (SDB) found that over half (116) of the 231 patients also complained of insomnia symptoms.[8] Since that time, additional studies have confirmed that insomnia and OSA co-occur more commonly than would be expected based on general population studies of each disorder separately.

Insomnia and OSA share several overlapping symptoms (**Fig. 1**), making an accurate diagnosis between insomnia, OSA, or COMISA more complicated and possibly confounding subsequent treatment approaches and decisions. There is evidence that adjunct assessment and management of comorbid insomnia in patients with COMISA can contribute to improved sleep, mental health, quality of life, and adherence to OSA therapy.[1,9–13] Therefore, it is important to identify and treat comorbid insomnia symptoms among patients seeking surgical options for OSA in the otolaryngology clinic setting.

CLINICAL RELEVANCE

OSA and Insomnia Have a Bidirectional Relationship

Insomnia and sleep apnea may have a reciprocal relationship in that 1 condition can worsen the other. For instance, the awakenings caused by sleep apnea can lead to difficulty falling back asleep, worsening insomnia symptoms. These repeated respiratory events and arousals promote a cardiorespiratory activation response that includes vasoconstriction, tachycardia, and hyperventilation.[14] During sleep, these responses can be highly alerting. Patients with OSA can also wake during an obstruction, as a combination of low lung volume, airway adhesion forces, and negative pressures below the site of obstruction requires significant neuromuscular effort to re-open the airway. This results in awakening while feeling a sensation of choking or gasping and can be particularly distressing. This feeling of distress may be more common in

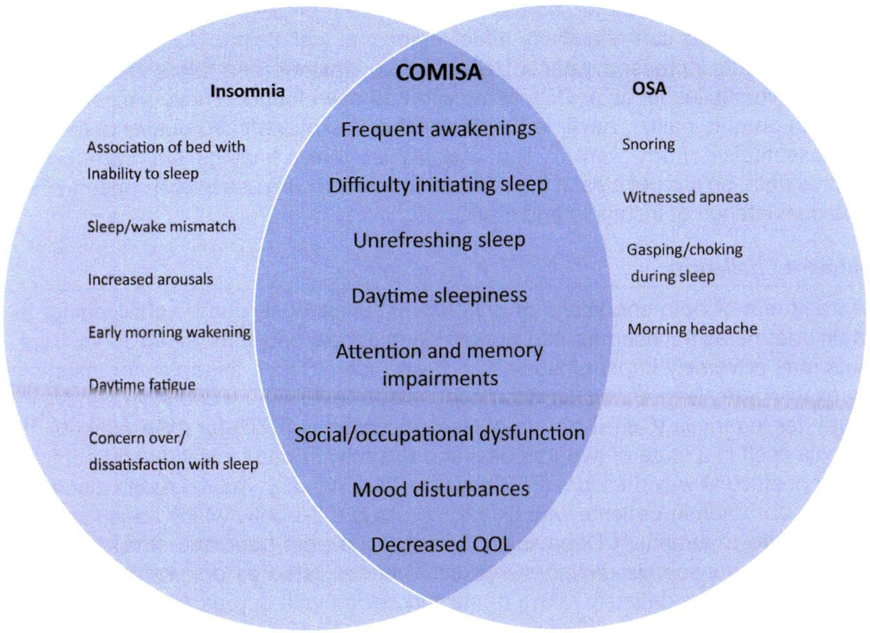

Fig. 1. Common symptoms in obstructive sleep apnea (OSA), insomnia, and co-morbid insomnia and OSA (COMISA). QOL, quality of life.

the phenotype of OSA with low respiratory arousal threshold (found in about one-third of OSA patients[3]), though studies of OSA phenotype in COMISA are lacking. The fragmentation of sleep that occurs in OSA also likely contributes to descriptions of non-restorative sleep and subsequent daytime impairments, which may culminate in patients reporting insomnia symptoms.[8,9] There is also evidence that insomnia may worsen OSA. Sleep fragmentation and sleep deprivation have been shown to increase the frequency and duration of obstructive respiratory events among healthy individuals as well as those with OSA.[15,16] While these studies experimentally restricted sleep, a causal effect of disrupted sleep on OSA severity may prove to be a pathway between insomnia and OSA. Finally, a case study of a 75-year old male treated with continuous positive airway pressure (CPAP) for OSA noted increased residual obstructive events during 2 periods of acute insomnia. This study highlights the possibility that difficulties initiating and/or maintaining sleep may have direct effects on respiratory stability.[17]

COMISA is Associated with Increased Adverse Health Outcomes

As our clinical understanding of the deleterious effects of COMISA increases, studies have begun to show that the morbidity associated with COMISA is greater than that of only insomnia or OSA.[18,19] Not surprisingly, COMISA patients experience greater daytime and quality of life impairments than those with either disorder alone.[8,20,21] Patients with COMISA may experience impairments secondary to the additive effects of the 2 disorders, or a more complex interrelationship between reduced sleep quality and quantity and cognitive misperceptions of the effects of sleep on daytime symptoms.[22] Both insomnia and OSA are also independently associated with hypertension and cardiovascular disease.[23–26] It is unclear whether there is an additive risk in patients with COMISA, but data taken from the Sleep Heart Health Study suggest that

COMISA does confer a larger increase in all-cause mortality.[27] Lastly, sleep disturbances in COMISA can negatively affect emotional well-being. COMISA has been associated with increased rates of depression, anxiety, and other mood disorders[8,28,29] versus insomnia or OSA alone and has been found to have a high association with chronic pain,[29] daytime functional impairment, reduced quality of life,[30,31] and absenteeism from work.[32] The majority of these findings are from cross-sectional data, so it is not clear if the increased morbidity is a cause or a consequence of the coexistence of insomnia and OSA.

Treatment Challenges

The treatment of both conditions of COMISA simultaneously can be challenging, as certain treatments for insomnia can worsen sleep apnea, and some sleep apnea treatments may adversely impact insomnia. For example, certain therapies for insomnia may exacerbate sleep apnea symptoms (eg, sleep restriction in cognitive behavioral therapy for insomnia [CBT-i] or use of benzodiazepines [BZD] for OSA patients.[33]). Insomnia itself is a state of hyperarousal and this may impede initiation and continuation of positive airway pressure (PAP) therapy.[9] Additionally, mental health disorders are more common in patients with COMISA versus OSA-only, which adds layers of complexity to treatment.[34] Depression, anxiety, and post-traumatic stress disorder (PTSD) all have insomnia-related sleep disturbances listed as diagnostic criteria in the DSM-V, such as difficulty falling or staying asleep with depression, and frequent awakenings and difficulty maintaining sleep with anxiety and PTSD.[35] It is important to consider all aspects of an individual's sleep and mental health when assessing which medications and therapies may be helpful in treating either or both OSA and insomnia when approaching patients with COMISA. Growing evidence demonstrates that multidisciplinary, combined treatment of insomnia and OSA results in greater improvements in both conditions than approaching each 1 in isolation.[36]

TREATMENT OF COMISA

Treatment of Insomnia in the Setting of COMISA

Treatment for insomnia generally falls into either cognitive or pharmacologic modes of therapy. CBT-i has gained significant attention over the past several decades as it has been demonstrated to be a highly effective treatment that focuses on a patient's maladaptive beliefs and aims to alter the conditioned insomnia response.[37,38] During weekly sessions, trained sleep therapists or psychologists utilize cognitive, behavioral, and psycho-educational tools to target the root causes leading to insomnia and mitigate anxiety about the sleep environment that contributes to prolonged arousals.[12] Recently, studies have compared groups of patients with COMISA or insomnia-only and found similar improvements in insomnia symptomatology after undergoing CBT-i.[12,39] Further evidence that CBT-i is efficacious in patients with COMISA was demonstrated in a study that compared groups of veterans with insomnia and mild OSA that did and did not receive CBT-i; those who received CBT-i had greater improvements in insomnia symptoms than those who did not.[39] Additionally, the benefits of CBT-i have the potential to be sustained in the long term given lasting improvements in sleep hygiene that result from therapy that persist after discontinuation of therapy. Currently, the most common recommendation for treatment of COMISA is to start CBT-i before initiating treatment of OSA.[36] The rationale for this order of treatment would be to target underlying insomnia symptoms to improve sleep onset and sleep efficiency, which would then ease the subsequent introduction and acceptance of a potentially disruptive treatment such as CPAP. Several challenges to usage of

CBT-i exist, however, such as its lack of widespread availability given the highly specialized personnel necessary for this therapy. Another barrier may be the sleep restriction that is commonly prescribed as a part of sleep retraining in CBT-i. Critics of CBT-i in patients with COMISA have raised the concern that worsening already present excessive daytime sleepiness may increase safety risks in these patients, such as motor vehicle accidents.[1] Despite these concerns, CBT-i is well accepted as a therapy for insomnia and its effectiveness in patients with COMISA continues to be demonstrated in a growing body of research.[12,36,40]

Pharmacologic therapy for insomnia, known as sedative-hypnotic medications, is also a mainstay of treatment for COMISA patients and typically targets sleep latency and sleep efficiency.[38] While efficacy of sleep aid medications is similar to behavioral therapy, there is a lack of evidence for pharmacologic treatment providing lasting changes to sleep hygiene and insomnia symptomatology once it is discontinued.[37] However, given its ready availability, pharmacologic treatment is currently more commonly utilized than CBT-i and its usage has become even more widespread as newer medications become available that minimize side effects of previous options. Melatonin and doxepin are often considered first-line treatment, particularly in older adults.[36] BZD and barbiturate drugs were commonly prescribed in the past and also have anxiolytic properties but have largely been abandoned as treatment for insomnia given the high risk of developing physical dependence and severe withdrawal symptoms after cessation.[38] Additionally, these medications can worsen OSA due to respiratory depression. For example, a triazolam dose of 0.25 mg has been shown to increase the duration of respiratory episodes in patients with known severe OSA and decrease the oxygen nadir and the arousal threshold after apneic events.[10] Non-BZD drugs, for example, the "z-drugs" (zolpidem, eszopiclone, and zaleplon), mediate sedation and amnesia and possess lesser, but still present, abuse potential. They have less impact on respiratory control mechanisms and have been shown to be of benefit in patients with COMISA, particularly in improving short-term adherence to CPAP therapy.[1,11,38] Lastly, a number of atypical antidepressant (eg, trazodone) and antipsychotic drugs (eg, olanzapine, quetiapine) have been noted to treat insomnia symptoms and are sometimes prescribed off-label. However, they are currently not recommended for insomnia unless being used to treat underlying mental health conditions.[38]

Treatment of OSA in the Setting of COMISA

CPAP has been considered first-line therapy for OSA for many decades and is highly efficacious when patients accept and comply with this treatment modality. However, insomnia can negatively affect CPAP compliance in patients with COMISA. For example, patients who experience difficulty with sleep initiation may also experience anticipatory anxiety related to mask discomfort which decreases their ability to use CPAP effectively. In addition, awakenings at night caused by discomfort with CPAP equipment or arousals due to residual OSA can be especially disruptive for patients with insomnia who already have a heightened tendency toward wakefulness.[1] In these cases, non-CPAP alternative treatments, including non-surgical and surgical options, eliminate the CPAP apparatus that can exacerbate existing issues with insomnia. One non-invasive treatment, the mandibular advancement device (MAD), has been shown to be helpful in patients with CPAP intolerance, particularly in patients with mild OSA.[41] While patients with COMISA utilizing MAD have not been widely studied, initial findings from a multi-center study comparing patients with COMISA and OSA-only who received MAD found that patients with COMISA had greater improvements in sleep latency compared to the OSA-only group.[42] These findings suggest that not only can MAD effectively treat certain patients with OSA, but it is possible that usage of MAD can also ameliorate insomnia in CPAP-intolerant patients with COMISA. Another option of pharmacologic treatment for OSA, the oral drug combination of atomoxetine and aroxybutynin (AD109), was recently introduced and is currently entering clinical trials. This treatment aims to activate upper airway muscles to maintain and open the airway during sleep and may ultimately be another option to treat patients with COMISA in the future if approved.[43]

Pharyngeal surgery has been a mainstay of surgical therapy for OSA since uvulopalatopharyngoplasty was introduced to North America in the 1980s by Fujita.[44] While pharyngeal procedures have shown limited efficacy without optimal patient selection, the static nature of changes as a result of healing provide a stable result when treating COMISA and any improvements in AHI may translate to greater sleep consolidation with possible improvement in sleep efficiency. Another promising surgical therapy with regard to COMISA is hypoglossal nerve stimulation (HGNS). Introduced in the United States in 2014, HGNS creates airway opening via tongue protrusion with each inspiration during sleep. While efficacy in terms of long-term AHI reduction in most patients receiving HGNS has been well established,[45,46] data in terms of insomnia outcomes are more limited, albeit promising. Although patients with COMISA have been shown to have poorer adherence to CPAP than those with OSA-only,[47–49] a recent study utilizing a large multicenter industry registry of patients receiving HGNS found that adherence was similar between COMISA and OSA-only groups. Additionally, postoperative insomnia scores as measured by the Insomnia Severity Index (ISI) improved to the greatest degree in patients with moderate-severe insomnia at baseline.[50] Another study found "meaningful improvements" in ISI score in 44% of patients with COMISA at 1 year follow-up, although this study was limited by small sample size.[51] It is possible that increased comfort with HGNS due to removal of the external apparatus of other devices may alleviate anxiety related to the ability to fall and stay asleep as well as ease sleep transitions.

SUMMARY

Patients with COMISA face challenges related to the synergism of insomnia and OSA that worsens physical, cognitive, and behavioral health compared to those with OSA alone. COMISA contributes to reduced sleep quality and is related to a high prevalence of psychiatric diseases which impact symptoms and treatment outcomes. Poor adherence to standard treatments for OSA such as CPAP must be identified and proactively addressed in patients with COMISA by treating insomnia with behavioral and/or pharmacologic therapies while also considering non-CPAP alternatives. In all patients with COMISA, multidisciplinary treatment is critical to address the complexities of these dual sleep disorders. Integration of care between sleep medicine, sleep surgery, mental and behavioral health, dentistry, primary care, and trained CBT-i providers with 1 service designated as central will help coordinate care and allow patients with COMISA to obtain optimal benefit from their chosen treatment. When considering sleep surgery, otolaryngologists must be aware that insomnia commonly co-occurs with OSA and be prepared to quantify its severity with tools such as the ISI in the same way that they measure OSA with polysomnography. Standardized preoperative counseling and intensive postoperative management to optimize healing with pharyngeal surgery and device usage after HGNS will be necessary to ensure the greatest health benefits from a surgical approach to OSA in patients with COMISA.

CLINICS CARE POINTS

- There is a high incidence of insomnia in patients with obstructive sleep apnea.
- Insomnia and obstructive sleep apnea appear to have a bidiractional relationship.
- Treatment for comorbid insomnia and obstructive sleep apnea can be challenging and should include a multi-disciplinary approach.
- Otolaryngologists should be prepared to characterize patients with comorbid insomnia to optimize patient care and improve clinical outcomes.

DISCLOSURE

Kathleen Sarber has no conflicts of interest to disclose. Reena Dhanda Patil has no conflicts of interest to disclose.

REFERENCES

1. Lack L, Sweetman A. Diagnosis and Treatment of Insomnia Comorbid with Obstructive Sleep Apnea. Sleep Med Clin 2016;11(3):379–88.
2. American Academy of Sleep Medicine. International classification of sleep disorders. American Academy of Sleep Medicine; 2014.
3. Eckert DJ. Phenotypic approaches to obstructive sleep apnoea - New pathways for targeted therapy. Sleep Med Rev 2018;37:45–59.
4. Guilleminault C, Eldridge FL, Dement WC. Insomnia with sleep apnea: a new syndrome. Science 1973;181(4102):856–8.
5. Peppard PE, Young T, Barnet JH, et al. Increased prevalence of sleep-disordered breathing in adults. Am J Epidemiol 2013;177(9):1006–14.
6. Ohayon MM. Epidemiology of insomnia: what we know and what we still need to learn. Sleep Med Rev 2002;6(2):97–111.
7. Lichstein KL, Riedel BW, Lester KW, et al. Occult sleep apnea in a recruited sample of older adults with insomnia. J Consult Clin Psychol 1999;67(3):405–10.
8. Krakow B, Melendrez D, Ferreira E, et al. Prevalence of insomnia symptoms in patients with sleep-disordered breathing. Chest 2001;120(6):1923–9.
9. Björnsdóttir E, Janson C, Sigurdsson JF, et al. Symptoms of insomnia among patients with obstructive sleep apnea before and after two years of positive airway pressure treatment. Sleep 2013;36(12):1901–9.
10. Berry RB, Kouchi K, Bower J, et al. Triazolam in patients with obstructive sleep apnea. Am J Respir Crit Care Med 1995;151(2 Pt 1):450–4.
11. Berry RB, Patel PB. Effect of zolpidem on the efficacy of continuous positive airway pressure as treatment for obstructive sleep apnea. Sleep 2006;29(8):1052–6.
12. Sweetman A, Lack L, Lambert S, et al. Does comorbid obstructive sleep apnea impair the effectiveness of cognitive and behavioral therapy for insomnia? Sleep Med 2017;39:38–46.
13. Sweetman A, Lack L, Bastien C. Co-Morbid Insomnia and Sleep Apnea (COMISA): Prevalence, Consequences, Methodological Considerations, and Recent Randomized Controlled Trials. Brain Sci 2019;9(12). https://doi.org/10.3390/brainsci9120371.
14. Younes M. Role of arousals in the pathogenesis of obstructive sleep apnea. Am J Respir Crit Care Med 2004;169(5):623–33.

15. Leiter JC, Knuth SL, Bartlett D Jr. The effect of sleep deprivation on activity of the genioglossus muscle. Am Rev Respir Dis 1985;132(6):1242–5.
16. Sériès F, Roy N, Marc I. Effects of sleep deprivation and sleep fragmentation on upper airway collapsibility in normal subjects. Am J Respir Crit Care Med 1994; 150(2):481–5.
17. Janssen HCJP, Venekamp LN, Peeters GAM, et al. Management of insomnia in sleep disordered breathing. Eur Respir Rev 2019;28(153). https://doi.org/10.1183/16000617.0080-2019.
18. Bianchi MT, Williams KL, McKinney S, et al. The subjective-objective mismatch in sleep perception among those with insomnia and sleep apnea. J Sleep Res 2013; 22(5):557–68.
19. Li Z, Li Y, Yang L, et al. Characterization of obstructive sleep apnea in patients with insomnia across gender and age. Sleep Breath 2015;19(2):723–7.
20. Björnsdóttir E, Janson C, Gíslason T, et al. Insomnia in untreated sleep apnea patients compared to controls. J Sleep Res 2012;21(2):131–8.
21. Smith S, Sullivan K, Hopkins W, et al. Frequency of insomnia report in patients with obstructive sleep apnoea hypopnea syndrome (OSAHS). Sleep Med 2004; 5(5):449–56.
22. Harvey AG. A cognitive model of insomnia. Behav Res Ther 2002;40(8):869–93.
23. Lanfranchi PA, Pennestri MH, Fradette L, et al. Nighttime blood pressure in normotensive subjects with chronic insomnia: implications for cardiovascular risk. Sleep 2009;32(6):760–6.
24. Bathgate CJ, Fernandez-Mendoza J. Insomnia, Short Sleep Duration, and High Blood Pressure: Recent Evidence and Future Directions for the Prevention and Management of Hypertension. Curr Hypertens Rep 2018;20(6):52.
25. Peppard PE, Young T, Palta M, et al. Prospective study of the association between sleep-disordered breathing and hypertension. N Engl J Med 2000; 342(19):1378–84.
26. O'Connor GT, Caffo B, Newman AB, et al. Prospective study of sleep-disordered breathing and hypertension: the Sleep Heart Health Study. Am J Respir Crit Care Med 2009;179(12):1159–64.
27. Lawton E, Jurisevic M, Hobart K, et al. P072 The Association Between Snoring and Hearing Loss in Patients with Obstructive Sleep Apnoea. Sleep Adv 2021; 2(Supplement_1):A44.
28. Lang CJ, Appleton SL, Vakulin A, et al. Co-morbid OSA and insomnia increases depression prevalence and severity in men. Respirology 2017;22(7):1407–15.
29. Krell SB, Kapur VK. Insomnia complaints in patients evaluated for obstructive sleep apnea. Sleep Breath 2005;9(3):104–10.
30. Stone J, Morin CM, Hart RP, et al. Neuropsychological functioning in older insomniacs with or without obstructive sleep apnea. Psychol Aging 1994;9(2):231–6.
31. Gooneratne NS, Gehrman PR, Nkwuo JE, et al. Consequences of comorbid insomnia symptoms and sleep-related breathing disorder in elderly subjects. Arch Intern Med 2006;166(16):1732–8.
32. Sivertsen B, Björnsdóttir E, Øverland S, et al. The joint contribution of insomnia and obstructive sleep apnoea on sickness absence. J Sleep Res 2013;22(2): 223–30.
33. Guilleminault C. Benzodiazepines, breathing, and sleep. Am J Med 1990;88(3A): 25S–8S.
34. Yang CM, Liao YS, Lin CM, et al. Psychological and behavioral factors in patients with comorbid obstructive sleep apnea and insomnia. J Psychosom Res 2011; 70(4):355–61.

35. Diagnostic and statistical manual of mental disorders: DSM-5-TR. American Psychiatric Association Publishing; 2022.
36. Sweetman AM, Lack LC, Catcheside PG, et al. Developing a successful treatment for co-morbid insomnia and sleep apnoea. Sleep Med Rev 2017;33:28–38.
37. Morin CM, Colecchi C, Stone J, et al. Behavioral and pharmacological therapies for late-life insomnia: a randomized controlled trial. JAMA 1999;281(11):991–9.
38. Matheson E, Hainer BL. Insomnia: Pharmacologic Therapy. Am Fam Physician 2017;96(1):29–35.
39. Fung CH, Martin JL, Josephson K, et al. Efficacy of Cognitive Behavioral Therapy for Insomnia in Older Adults With Occult Sleep-Disordered Breathing. Psychosom Med 2016;78(5):629–39.
40. Morin CM, Vallières A, Guay B, et al. Cognitive behavioral therapy, singly and combined with medication, for persistent insomnia: a randomized controlled trial. JAMA 2009;301(19):2005–15.
41. Marklund M, Franklin KA. Long-term effects of mandibular repositioning appliances on symptoms of sleep apnoea. J Sleep Res 2007;16(4):414–20.
42. Meira e Cruz M, Giannasi L, Machado M, et al. Management of comorbid insomnia and sleep apnea with mandibular advancement devices: first results from a multi-centric case-control study on the therapeutic outcomes. Sleep Med 2022;S257–8.
43. Schweitzer P, Ojile JM, Thein S, et al. The Oral Agent AD109 Improves Objective and Subjective Outcomes in Obstructive Sleep Apnea Patients. Results From the Mariposa Study, a Randomized, Controlled Clinical Trial. In: *A18. Breaking NEWS IN OSA: NEW approaches and NEW TRIALS*. American Thoracic Society International conference Abstracts. American Thoracic Society; 2023. p. A1052.
44. Fujita S, Conway W, Zorick F, et al. Surgical Correction of Anatomic Abnormalities in Obstructive Sleep Apnea Syndrome: Uvulopalatopharyngoplasty. Otolaryngol Head Neck Surg 1981;89(6):923–34.
45. Thaler E, Schwab R, Maurer J, et al. Results of the ADHERE upper airway stimulation registry and predictors of therapy efficacy. Laryngoscope 2020;130(5):1333–8.
46. Woodson BT, Soose RJ, Gillespie MB, et al. Three-Year Outcomes of Cranial Nerve Stimulation for Obstructive Sleep Apnea: The STAR Trial. Otolaryngol Head Neck Surg 2016;154(1):181–8.
47. Wickwire EM, Smith MT, Birnbaum S, et al. Sleep maintenance insomnia complaints predict poor CPAP adherence: A clinical case series. Sleep Med 2010;11(8):772–6.
48. Wallace DM, Sawyer AM, Shafazand S. Comorbid insomnia symptoms predict lower 6-month adherence to CPAP in US veterans with obstructive sleep apnea. Sleep Breath 2018;22(1):5–15.
49. Bahr K, Cámara RJA, Gouveris H, et al. Current Treatment of Comorbid Insomnia and Obstructive Sleep Apnea With CBTI and PAP-Therapy: A Systematic Review. Front Neurol 2018;9:804.
50. Dhanda Patil R, Ishman SL, Chang JL, et al. Impact of Insomnia on Hypoglossal Nerve Stimulation Outcomes in the ADHERE Registry. Laryngoscope 2023. https://doi.org/10.1002/lary.30933.
51. Pieh C, Bach M, Popp R, et al. Insomnia symptoms influence CPAP compliance. Sleep Breath 2013;17(1):99–104.

Management of Obstructive Sleep Apnea in the Infant and Newborn

Jillian N. Sanford, MD[a], Derek J. Lam, MD, MPH[b,*]

KEYWORDS

• Pediatric • Obstructive sleep apnea • Sleep disordered breathing • Infant • Neonate • Laryngomalacia • CPAP • Micrognathia

KEY POINTS

- Obstructive sleep apnea in infants is less well defined than in older age groups with distinct features of sleep physiology that are different than in older children.
- Etiologies of upper airway obstruction in infants and newborns are varied and often related to congenital anatomic problems like choanal atresia, micrognathia, or laryngomalacia.
- Laryngomalacia is the most common cause of airway obstruction and obstructive sleep apnea in infants and can usually be treated with either observation or supraglottoplasty.

INTRODUCTION

Obstructive sleep apnea (OSA) is common in children with estimated prevalence of 1% to 6%.[1] However, infants and neonates represent a unique population where age-specific norms for polysomnography (PSG) are less well defined than other age groups, and prevalence remains unknown. Similarly, while adenotonsillectomy is the recognized first-line treatment for OSA in children ages 2 years and older, tonsillar hypertrophy is much less common among infants less than 1 year of age.[2] In this age group, any upper airway obstruction that impacts respiration during wakefulness can also cause sleep-disordered breathing or OSA, and it is often multifactorial in etiology. Infant airways are more prone to collapse and obstruction due to congenital craniofacial anomalies, laryngeal or tracheal anomalies, immature pharyngeal dilator muscles, greater chest wall compliance, poor ventilatory control, and the laryngeal chemoreflex leading to laryngospasm. Therefore, both diagnostic and treatment

[a] Division of Pediatric Pulmonology and Sleep Medicine, Department of Pediatrics, Oregon Health and Science University, 3181 Southwest Sam Jackson Park Road, Portland, OR 97239, USA; [b] Pediatric Otolaryngology Division, Department of Otolaryngology–Head and Neck Surgery, Oregon Health and Science University, 3181 Southwest Sam Jackson Park Road, Portland, OR 97239, USA
* Corresponding author.
E-mail address: lamde@ohsu.edu

Otolaryngol Clin N Am 57 (2024) 395–405
https://doi.org/10.1016/j.otc.2024.02.006
0030-6665/24/

strategies for OSA differ significantly in infants compared to older children. Owing to a lack of consensus guidelines for the management of OSA in infants, the treatment approach for OSA in infants is largely a product of clinician experience, caregiver preference, and symptom severity. Treatment decisions may be complicated by a variety of other factors including distance to sleep center, caregiver capability, and family circumstances. A multidisciplinary approach involving pediatric sleep medicine, otolaryngology, neonatology, pulmonology, craniofacial surgery, and genetics is often required, depending on the comorbidities and medical complexity of the child.

DIAGNOSIS

Identifying infants at risk for OSA requires taking a thoughtful clinical history, including consideration of comorbidities. Snoring is a common and well-known clinical symptom of OSA, but is less reliable in this age group given that infants without OSA may snore (11.8%–26% of infants snore, but <10% of snoring infants have OSA).[3] Furthermore, other at-risk groups of infants, including those with micrognathia or cleft palate, often do not snore. Caregivers and/or health care providers may report observation of pauses in breathing, history of brief respiratory unexplained event, failure to thrive, insomnia, family history of OSA, or hypoxemia during sleep. Physical examination during wakefulness may be normal or yield findings of noisy breathing, hypotonia, tonsillar hypertrophy, or features related to other medical disorders or syndromes. Diagnostic PSG should be considered in these infants, and those with other known risk factors including prematurity, craniofacial disorders, history of prematurity, neurologic disorders, Down syndrome, and other genetic conditions (**Box 1**).

There are no universally accepted guidelines for the diagnosis and management of OSA in infants even though diagnostic PSG is widely touted as the gold standard for diagnosis of OSA in children. However, testing infants is resource intensive and may not be readily available outside of academic centers due to the need for a dedicated sleep technologist for the infant being evaluated (1:1 ratio), and few labs with staff or

Box 1
Comorbidities associated with obstructive sleep in infants

Gastroesophageal reflux

Prematurity (<32 weeks gestation)

Achondroplasia

Beckwith–Wiedemann syndrome

Bronchopulmonary dysplasia associated with prematurity

Craniofacial disorders
- Pierre Robin Sequence
- Syndromic craniosynostosis (Apert, Crouzon, Pfeiffer, Saethre-Chotzen syndromes)
- Treacher-Collins
- Hemifacial microsomia

Down syndrome

Hypotonia, including cerebral palsy

Chiari malformation

Mucopolysaccharidoses

Prader–Willi syndrome

pediatric sleep providers trained to perform and interpret infant sleep testing. There is increasing interest in using pulse oximetry to aid in the diagnosis of OSA in children, but there is limited evidence, especially in infants. Portable overnight pulse oximetry has demonstrated a high sensitivity and positive predictive value for OSA and may be a useful screening tool to identify infants at risk for more severe OSA, but a normal oximetry study cannot exclude OSA. For infants with a strong clinical suspicion or high risk for OSA, confirmatory diagnostic PSG is needed to establish the diagnosis and severity of disease.[4] Despite the fact that portable home oximetry is thought to be easily accessible, it is also precarious and prone to accidental removal by the patient or suboptimal placement by the caregiver.

Pathophysiological and practical differences exist between infants and older children: infants have increased upper airway and chest wall compliance, relative ventilatory instability with increased propensity for central apneas, laryngeal chemoreflex (glottic closure due to reflux or aspiration), spend more time in rapid eye movement sleep, and less consolidated nighttime sleep with increased arousals. Given these differences, PSGs in healthy term neonates and infants show reasonably elevated respiratory indices (overall apnea–hypopnea index [AHI], obstructive AHI [oAHI], and/or central apnea index) and there is concern that using standard pediatric diagnostic cutoffs, even in at-risk infants, may prompt clinicians to pursue overly aggressive treatments for otherwise physiologic findings (**Table 1**).

The American Academy of Pediatrics Clinical Practice Guideline on the Diagnosis and Management of Childhood OSA Syndrome explicitly excludes infants younger than 1 year of age and recommends consultation with a pediatric subspecialist.[1] However, the European Respiratory Society Task Force published a statement in 2017 on obstructive sleep-disordered breathing in 1 to 23 month old children, stating that infants are frequently diagnosed using standard pediatric cutoffs (mild OSA defined as oAHI 1–5/hour, moderate OSA as 5–10/h, severe as more than 10/h).[5] Owing to the lack of consensus, there is significant variability in clinician practice patterns. When anonymously surveyed through PEDSLEEP and Ped-Lung Listservs, a group of 54 providers from 8 countries report using different obstructive AHI cutoffs to make the diagnosis of OSA in infants, with additional variation attributed to subgroups (neonates, younger infants, and older infants)[6] (**Fig. 1**).

Early identification and treatment of OSA in children is important to prevent neurocognitive dysfunction, but the long-term outcomes of untreated OSA in infants are unknown. Further research is needed to define normative data in infants, cutoffs for the diagnosis of OSA, and parameters to inform treatment plans that include an emphasis on longitudinal outcomes.

ETIOLOGY OF OBSTRUCTIVE SLEEP APNEA IN INFANTS

The etiology of OSA in infants is multifactorial and often a product of one or more of the following: differences in the bony scaffold of the upper airway, frequently involving micrognathia, neuromuscular hypotonia, soft tissue obstruction or other congenital abnormality, and increased loop gain/immature control of breathing.

Nasal Obstruction

Because neonates are obligate nasal breathers, infants with nasal obstruction may present with chronic respiratory distress including noisy (stertorous) breathing with cyclical cyanosis that is relieved by crying and worse during feeding. Nasal obstruction is suspected as a contributor to such distress when there is an inability to pass a 5/6 Fr suction catheter through one or both sides of the nasal airway. The most

Table 1
Comparison of reference values for apnea–hypopnea index, obstructive apnea hypopnea index, and central apnea index from various studies that recruited healthy infants and used AASM Scoring rules[40]

Authors (Methods)	Age Groups <1 mo	1 mo	3 mo	12 mo
Daftary et al,[41] 2019 (Nocturnal PSG)	AHI 14.5/h (1–37.7) CAI 3.3/h (0–27.2)			
Kanack et al,[42] 2022 (Nap PSG)	AHI 6.9/h (2–23) Obstructive AHI 4.9/h (1.7–19.1) CAI 0.7/h (0.0–12.4)			
Brocmann et al,[43] 2013 (Nocturnal polygraphy)		AHI 7.8/h (95th percentile 25.5/h) Obstructive AHI 1.5/h (95th percentile 5.8/h) CAI 5.5/h (95th percentile 20.5/h)	AHI 4.9/h (95th percentile 26.4/h) Obstructive AHI 0.9/h (95th percentile 3.4/h) CAI 4.1/h (95th percentile 24.2/h)	
Vezina et al,[44] 2020 (Nocturnal polygraphy)				AHI 4.2/h (90th percentile 10.7/h) CAI 2.5/h (90th percentile 7.1/h)

Results are presented as median (range) or median (90th or 95th percentile).
Abbreviation: CAI, central apnea index.
From Kaditis A, Gozal D. Sleep Studies for Clinical Indications during the First Year of Life: Infants Are Not Small Children Children (Basel). 2022 Apr; 9(4): 523.Published online 2022 Apr 7. https://doi.org/10.3390/children9040523.

common cause of nasal obstruction in a neonate is neonatal rhinitis, a common newborn condition characterized by clear or mucoid discharge with nasal mucosal edema in an otherwise healthy newborn. It is considered a physiologic condition with exaggerated parasympathetic response including local inflammatory mediators often implicated in allergic conditions. These patients will lack a clinical history of infectious or anatomic cause and may be treated conservatively with nasal steroid drops (generally used with preceding nasal saline and suction), or nasal decongestants like oxymetazoline or neosynephrine.

Congenital bony abnormalities like pyriform aperture stenosis or choanal atresia are rarer conditions, but can cause severe respiratory distress during both wakefulness and sleep. Congenital nasal pyriform aperture stenosis (CNPAS) is estimated to occur in only 1 in 25,000 live births. It is characterized by a bony overgrowth of the nasal

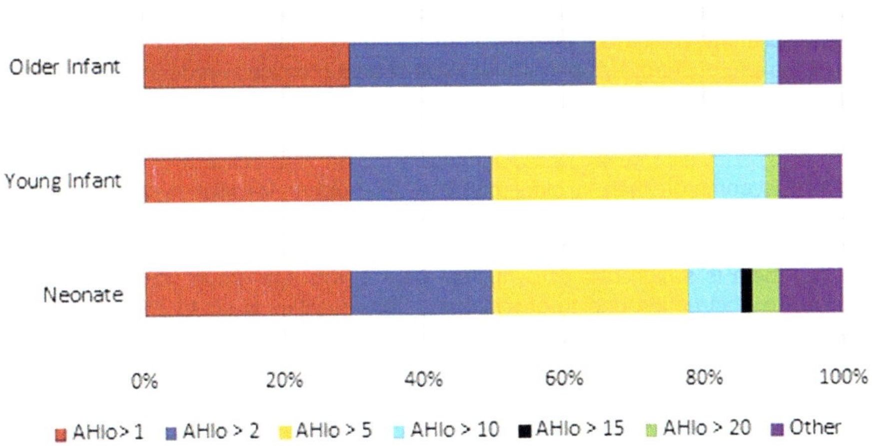

Fig. 1. oAHI cutoff for OSA diagnosis. oAHI, obstructive apnea-hypopnea index; OSA, obstructive sleep apnea. (*From* Kombathula R, Ingram DG, Ehsan Z. Current Practice Patterns in the Diagnosis and Management of Sleep-Disordered Breathing in Infants. J Clin Sleep Med. Oct 15 2019;15(10):1427-1431. https://doi.org/10.5664/jcsm.7968.)

process of the maxilla and is typically diagnosed radiographically using noncontrast axial computed tomographic (CT) imaging. A nasal pyriform aperture width of less than 11 mm in a term infant is considered diagnostic of CNPAS.[7] It is thought to be a microform of holoprosencephaly and is associated with other midline abnormalities such as a single central maxillary incisor, so any infant diagnosed with CNPAS should have brain CT and MRI and spine radiography to screen for other midline defects. Mild cases of CNPAS can be treated medically with nasal decongestants or topical corticosteroids as in neonatal rhinitis. More severe cases that do not respond to this medical treatment (usually with a pyriform aperture width < 6 mm) are treated surgically through a sublabial incision and resection of the inferolateral bone of the pyriform aperture using a drill.[8,9]

Choanal atresia occurs with an incidence between 1 in 5000 and 1 in 8000 live births and is often associated with an underlying syndrome such as CHARGE association. It occurs as a mixed bony/membranous atresia in 70% and a pure bony atresia in 30% of cases and can be unilateral (60%) or bilateral (40%).[10] Like CNPAS, the diagnosis is confirmed radiographically using axial CT images or endoscopically with rigid or flexible nasendoscopy. Bilateral choanal atresia is usually diagnosed early in the neonatal period due to the significant respiratory distress and cyclic cyanosis associated with an inability to breathe through the nose, and requires early surgical correction in the first few weeks of life in order to stabilize the infant airway. This is most often performed through a transnasal endoscopic approach with either microdebrider or puncture and dilation, though transpalatal approaches have also been described.[11] Unilateral choanal atresia is less symptomatic and the diagnosis can often be missed until the child is older. Even if appropriately diagnosed, definitive repair is often delayed until 2 to 3 years of age when the repair is technically easier and there is less risk of complications or recurrent stenosis. Postoperative stenting using trimmed endotracheal tubes for variable durations from 5 days to several weeks has been reported, most often in cases of syndromic bilateral choanal atresia such as in CHARGE association, but it remains unclear whether stenting substantially improves the rate of restenosis.[11] Multiple revisions to address restenosis are common, especially in cases of bilateral syndromic choanal atresia, with one study reporting a mean of 5.24 operations for bilateral versus 2.2 operations for unilateral choanal atresia.[12] Recent reports of the use of steroid-eluting stents have shown promise in reducing the rate of restenosis and need for revision procedures.[13]

Adenotonsillar Hypertrophy

Though less common than in older children, adenoid or tonsillar hypertrophy has been reported as contributors to OSA in infants, and adenotonsillectomy has been shown to improve OSA severity in a majority of children aged less than 3 years.[14] However, there is a high rate of persistent OSA in this age group which has been attributed to obstruction due to other airway abnormalities in up to 73% of infants aged less than 18 months, such as laryngomalacia, subglottic stenosis, or tracheobronchomalacia.[15] In addition, there is a greater risk of perioperative complications in this age group with respect to respiratory distress, hemorrhage, and poor oral intake.[16] For this reason, overnight inpatient observation is recommended for children aged less than 3 years.[17] Adenoidectomy alone is more commonly performed in children aged less than 2 years than in older children, and a recent systematic review demonstrated the greatest impact in children less than 12 months old (95% reduction in AHI).[18]

Micrognathia

Patients with micrognathia may be thought of along a spectrum, with mild isolated nonsyndromic micrognathia often resolving spontaneously and more complex syndromic cases typically necessitating medical or surgical intervention. Conservative management includes prone positioning and nasopharyngeal stenting.[19] The use of prone positioning must be balanced with the risk of sudden unexpected infant death syndrome[20] and patients are routinely monitored with continuous pulse oximetry while prone to mitigate this risk. Infants with severe micrognathia resulting in glossoptosis and upper airway obstruction, the definition of Pierre Robin Sequence (PRS), can sometimes be adequately managed with these conservative measures, but often require prolonged treatment or more definitive surgical management.[21] Infants with syndromic PRS, as in Stickler syndrome or 22q11 deletion syndrome, are not expected to have normal mandibular growth after birth due to their underlying genetic growth disturbance.[22] Positional therapy has been reported successful in improving airway obstruction in 50% of infants with syndromic PRS, compared to 72% of infants with nonsyndromic PRS,[23] highlighting that multiple mechanisms, including impaired upper airway motor control may also play a role. Roughly one-third of infants with PRS who fail to respond sufficiently to positional therapy will respond to nasopharyngeal stenting, which is accomplished through transnasal placement of a standard 3.0 or 3.5 sized endotracheal tube to the level of the hypopharynx.[24] While effective, the downsides to this treatment include inability for the infant to feed and need for the routine replacement of the nasopharyngeal stent every 4 to 6 weeks. Both positional therapy and nasopharyngeal stenting are considered temporizing measures to manage symptoms while awaiting mandibular growth, but the duration of such treatment can vary considerably, sometimes lasting for months.

In severe cases where surgical intervention is being considered, airway evaluation in the form of direct laryngoscopy and bronchoscopy is recommended to assess the ease and stability of intubation, and to evaluate for other airway pathology that may alter the treatment plan. Awake nasopharyngoscopy or drug-induced sleep endoscopy can also help to gauge the severity of glossoptosis and airway stability in the absence of rigid instrumentation.[25] Whenever possible, PSG is recommended to characterize the severity of obstruction and help guide clinical decision-making.[26] Severe OSA might prompt more aggressive intervention than milder disease where conservative methods could be used as temporizing measures to allow for growth and gradual improvement over time. When obstructive symptoms are severe even when awake or when PSG demonstrates severe OSA, surgical treatment should be considered. Mandibular distraction osteogenesis (MDO) can be performed during the neonatal period in both syndromic and nonsyndromic PRS, and high rates of success in avoiding tracheotomy have been reported.[27] A recent study demonstrated that MDO can successfully treat severe OSA in the neonatal period with improvement in the median oAHI from 33 to 6.8 events hour.[28] However, not all infants with PRS can be successfully treated with MDO. For example, severely afflicted syndromic patients with insufficient mandibular bone have demonstrated lower success rates.[29,30] In such cases, or where MDO fails to adequately relieve the upper airway obstruction, tracheotomy is a definitive treatment for both airway stability and OSA.

Laryngomalacia

Laryngomalacia is the most common cause of stridor and OSA in infants. It is characterized by intermittent obstruction of the laryngeal inlet due to prolapse of the arytenoid cartilage and its mucosa anteriorly, often in combination with lateral curling or retroflexion of an omega-shaped epiglottis. Symptoms include stridor during wakefulness that is worst with agitation or feeding, but it can also cause OSA in infants and has been implicated as a cause of sudden infant death syndrome. This form of laryngomalacia that primarily affects infants is referred to as congenital laryngomalacia and can be distinguished from sleep-dependent laryngomalacia where the symptoms of stridor and obstruction occur only during sleep and not during wakefulness. Sleep-dependent laryngomalacia is diagnosed with drug-induced sleep endoscopy rather than awake nasopharyngoscopy and typically occurs in older children (>2 years old) and those with comorbidities like Down syndrome or hypotonia.

Infants with mild presentation (mild intermittent stridor without significant increased work of breathing during wakefulness or sleep, adequate feeding, and good weight gain) or mild OSA based on PSG can often be managed with periodic monitoring over the first 1 to 2 years of life. Gastroesophageal reflux is often associated with laryngomalacia in infants, and mild symptoms or OSA severity can sometimes be treated with acid suppression medication.[31] Though traditionally diagnosed and treated based on the severity of stridor and feeding difficulty during wakefulness, PSG or nocturnal pulse oximetry has increasingly been used to help define the severity of disease and aid in the decision to recommend surgical intervention.[4,32] In practice, there is a very high rate of diagnosing OSA in infants with symptomatic laryngomalacia,[32–34] often prompting surgical intervention even when symptoms are relatively mild and observation with eventual spontaneous resolution could occur. This was observed in a recent study examining changes over time observed on PSG in infants treated with supraglottoplasty and those who were just observed. They noted no significant differences in the mean age at resolution of OSA between the two groups (35 vs 42 months, respectively, $P=.60$), though they did note that infants with other comorbidities like neurologic disease or genetic syndromes did require significantly more time for the OSA to resolve.[35] Thus, the utility of PSG in the diagnosis and management of symptomatic laryngomalacia remains controversial. Nevertheless, supraglottoplasty has been shown to be effective in treating laryngomalacia, whether assessed by awake symptoms of stridor and feeding difficulty, weight gain, or by PSG. Two recent meta-analyses of the impact of supraglottoplasty demonstrated oAHI reductions of approximately 20 events per hour but with a high rate of persistent OSA

(73%–88%), based on studies with heterogeneous patient populations, though mostly comprised infants in the first year of life.[36,37]

SUPPLEMENTAL OXYGEN AND POSITIVE AIRWAY PRESSURE

It is not known whether high flow nasal cannula is effective in the treatment of OSA in infants. However, low flow supplemental oxygen via nasal cannula and PAP therapy may be considered as a bridge therapy to offer time for growth while awaiting definitive corrective surgical intervention, or for long-term use depending on the long-term goals of care and the infant's other medical comorbidities. PAP therapy may successfully treat sleep-disordered breathing in infants, but adherence may be variable due to intolerance of pressure and nasal mask discomfort. Caregiver participation is required to comfort the infant and reposition the cannula or mask when needed. Oxygen therapy may be started empirically, but the infant will generally require an in-lab pulse oximetry titration. This follow-up sleep study will test different oxygen flow rates and ensure there is improvement in obstructive breathing events and oxygen saturation, without the development of hypoventilation. Other infants will be prescribed supplemental oxygen and/or PAP therapy following in laboratory testing which may include pulse oximetry titration, PAP titration study (CPAP or bi-level-PAP), or PAP titration study with supplemental oxygen therapy (requires both therapies). Most infants are prescribed home ventilators to deliver CPAP, due to lack of FDA approval for traditional CPAP machines in children who weigh less than 13 kg. These devices are more expensive and may limit access to treatment. In 2022, the American Academy of Sleep Medicine released a position statement that states CPAP can be a safe and effective outpatient treatment for children of younger ages and lower weights when managed by a clinician with expertise in evaluating and managing pediatric OSA.[38] Clinicians are hopeful this position will lead to practice change. Adherence data for infant use of PAP therapy are not well described in the literature, but young age was associated with acceptable CPAP adherence in children with OSA in a 2023 meta-analysis that evaluated for predictors of CPAP adherence in children with OSA.[39]

SUMMARY

OSA in infants presents a unique clinical challenge. The indications and interpretation of PSG are not well established in this population. Etiologies of OSA in this age group are varied and often associated with congenital anatomic anomalies that require different management strategies than in older children. This often requires multidisciplinary collaboration for optimal outcomes that could include surgical, medical, or combinations of treatments.

CLINICS CARE POINTS

- Obstructive sleep apnea should be considered in any infant with a history of noisy breathing or obstructive symptoms during wakefulness.
- Polysomnography results should be interpreted with caution due to physiologic features in infants that may predispose to elevated respiratory indices.
- Conservative medical treatment such as prone positioning, nasopharyngeal stenting, supplemental oxygen, or PAP therapy can be used as bridge therapies, but definitive management often requires surgery targeting the specific anatomic causes of obstruction.

DISCLOSURE

The authors have nothing to disclose.

FUNDING

Dr Lam has two grants through NHLBI:R61HL165345 and R61HL162771.

REFERENCES

1. Marcus CL, Brooks LJ, Draper KA, et al. Diagnosis and management of childhood obstructive sleep apnea syndrome. Pediatrics 2012;130(3):e714–55.
2. Rayasam S, Johnson R, Lenahan D, et al. Obstructive Sleep Apnea in Children Under 3 Years of Age. Laryngoscope 2021;131(9):E2603–8.
3. Montgomery-Downs HE, Gozal D. Sleep habits and risk factors for sleep-disordered breathing in infants and young toddlers in Louisville, Kentucky. Sleep Med 2006;7(3):211–9.
4. Makhout S, Boudewyns A, Van Hoorenbeeck K, et al. Nocturnal pulse oximetry as a possible screening method for obstructive sleep apnea in infants with laryngomalacia. Sleep Med 2022;90:91–5.
5. Kaditis AG, Alonso Alvarez ML, Boudewyns A, et al. ERS statement on obstructive sleep disordered breathing in 1- to 23-month-old children. Eur Respir J 2017;50(6).
6. Kombathula R, Ingram DG, Ehsan Z. Current Practice Patterns in the Diagnosis and Management of Sleep-Disordered Breathing in Infants. J Clin Sleep Med 2019;15(10):1427–31.
7. Belden CJ, Mancuso AA, Schmalfuss IM. CT features of congenital nasal piriform aperture stenosis: initial experience. Radiology 1999;213(2):495–501.
8. Chakravarty PD, Sim F, Slim MAM, et al. Congenital nasal pyriform aperture stenosis; our experience of 34 cases. Int J Pediatr Otorhinolaryngol 2023;166:111491.
9. Wormald R, Hinton-Bayre A, Bumbak P, et al. Congenital nasal pyriform aperture stenosis 5.7 mm or less is associated with surgical intervention: A pooled case series. Int J Pediatr Otorhinolaryngol 2015;79(11):1802–5.
10. Ramsden JD, Campisi P, Forte V. Choanal atresia and choanal stenosis. Otolaryngol Clin North Am 2009;42(2):339–52, x.
11. Gundle L, Ojha S, Hendry J, et al. Stenting versus stentless repair for bilateral choanal atresia: A systematic review of the literature. Int J Pediatr Otorhinolaryngol 2021;151:110926.
12. Attya H, Callaby M, Thevasagayam R. Choanal atresia surgery: outcomes in 42 patients over 20 years and a review of the literature. Eur Arch Oto-Rhino-Laryngol 2021;278(7):2347–56.
13. Wilcox LJ, Smith MM, de Alarcon A, et al. Use of Steroid-Eluting Stents after Endoscopic Repair of Choanal Atresia: A Case Series with Review. Ann Otol Rhinol Laryngol 2020;129(10):1003–10.
14. Rayasam SS, Abijay C, Johnson R, et al. Outcomes of adenotonsillectomy for obstructive sleep apnea in children under 3 years of age. Ear Nose Throat J 2022. 1455613221086526.
15. Rastatter JC, Schroeder JW Jr, French A, et al. Synchronous airway lesions in children younger than age 3 years undergoing adenotonsillectomy. Otolaryngol Head Neck Surg 2011;145(2):309–13.
16. Cooper F, Spektor Z, Kay DJ. Rate and risk factors for post-adenotonsillectomy complications in children under 24 months and 24 to 36 months old. Am J Otolaryngol 2020;41(4):102546.

17. Mitchell RB, Archer SM, Ishman SL, et al. Clinical Practice Guideline: Tonsillectomy in Children (Update). Otolaryngol Head Neck Surg 2019;160(1_suppl):S1–42.
18. Reckley LK, Song SA, Chang ET, et al. Adenoidectomy can improve obstructive sleep apnoea in young children: systematic review and meta-analysis. J Laryngol Otol 2016;130(11):990–4.
19. Evans KN, Sie KC, Hopper RA, et al. Robin sequence: from diagnosis to development of an effective management plan. Pediatrics 2011;127(5):936–48.
20. Greenlee CJ, Scholes MA, Gao D, et al. Obstructive Sleep Apnea and Sleep Position: Does It Matter for Infants With a Cleft Palate? Cleft Palate Craniofac J 2019; 56(7):890–5.
21. Meyer AC, Lidsky ME, Sampson DE, et al. Airway interventions in children with Pierre Robin Sequence. Otolaryngol Head Neck Surg 2008;138(6):782–7.
22. Mackay DR. Controversies in the diagnosis and management of the Robin sequence. J Craniofac Surg 2011;22(2):415–20.
23. Smith MC, Senders CW. Prognosis of airway obstruction and feeding difficulty in the Robin sequence. Int J Pediatr Otorhinolaryngol 2006;70(2):319–24.
24. Parhizkar N, Saltzman B, Grote K, et al. Nasopharyngeal airway for management of airway obstruction in infants with micrognathia. Cleft Palate Craniofac J 2011; 48(4):478–82.
25. de Sousa TV, Marques IL, Carneiro AF, et al. Nasopharyngoscopy in Robin sequence: clinical and predictive value. Cleft Palate Craniofac J 2003;40(6): 618–23.
26. Morrison KA, Collares MV, Flores RL. Robin Sequence: Neonatal Mandibular Distraction. Clin Plast Surg 2021;48(3):363–73.
27. Ow AT, Cheung LK. Meta-analysis of mandibular distraction osteogenesis: clinical applications and functional outcomes. Plast Reconstr Surg 2008;121(3): 54e–69e.
28. Kochhar R, Modi V, de Silva N, et al. Polysomnography-guided mandibular distraction osteogenesis in Pierre Robin sequence patients. J Clin Sleep Med 2022;18(7):1749–55.
29. Lam DJ, Tabangin ME, Shikary TA, et al. Outcomes of Mandibular Distraction Osteogenesis in the Treatment of Severe Micrognathia. JAMA otolaryngology– head & neck surgery 2014. https://doi.org/10.1001/jamaoto.2014.16.
30. Mandell DL, Yellon RF, Bradley JP, et al. Mandibular distraction for micrognathia and severe upper airway obstruction. Arch Otolaryngol Head Neck Surg 2004; 130(3):344–8.
31. Dobbie AM, White DR. Laryngomalacia. Pediatr Clin North Am 2013;60(4): 893–902.
32. Weinstein JE, Lawlor CM, Wu EL, et al. Utility of polysomnography in determination of laryngomalacia severity. Int J Pediatr Otorhinolaryngol 2017;93:145–9.
33. Fard D, Rohlfing ML, Razak A, et al. Prevalence and natural history of obstructive sleep apnea in pediatric patients with laryngomalacia. Int J Pediatr Otorhinolaryngol 2020;133:109967.
34. Verkest V, Verhulst S, Van Hoorenbeeck K, et al. Prevalence of obstructive sleep apnea in children with laryngomalacia and value of polysomnography in treatment decisions. Int J Pediatr Otorhinolaryngol 2020;137:110255.
35. Ratanakorn W, Brockbank J, Ishman S, et al. The maturation changes of sleep-related respiratory abnormalities in infants with laryngomalacia. J Clin Sleep Med 2021;17(4):767–77.

36. Farhood Z, Ong AA, Nguyen SA, et al. Objective Outcomes of Supraglottoplasty for Children With Laryngomalacia and Obstructive Sleep Apnea: A Meta-analysis. JAMA otolaryngology– head & neck surgery 2016;142(7):665–71.
37. Camacho M, Dunn B, Torre C, et al. Supraglottoplasty for laryngomalacia with obstructive sleep apnea: A systematic review and meta-analysis. Laryngoscope 2016;126(5):1246–55.
38. Amos L, Afolabi-Brown O, Gault D, et al. Age and weight considerations for the use of continuous positive airway pressure therapy in pediatric populations: an American Academy of Sleep Medicine position statement. J Clin Sleep Med 2022;18(8):2041–3.
39. Sawunyavisuth B, Ngamjarus C, Sawanyawisuth K. Adherence to Continuous Positive Airway Pressure Therapy in Pediatric Patients with Obstructive Sleep Apnea: A Meta-Analysis. Ther Clin Risk Manag 2023;19:143–62.
40. Kaditis A, Gozal D. Sleep Studies for Clinical Indications during the First Year of Life: Infants Are Not Small Children. Children (Basel) 2022;9(4):523.
41. Daftary AS, Jalou HE, Shively L, et al. Polysomnography Reference Values in Healthy Newborns. J Clin Sleep Med 2019;15(3):437–43.
42. Kanack MD, Nakra N, Ahmad I, Vyas RM. Normal Neonatal Sleep Defined: Refining Patient Selection and Interpreting Sleep Outcomes for Mandibular Distraction. Plast Reconstr Surg Glob Open 2022;10(1):e4031.
43. Brockmann PE, Poets A, Poets CF. Reference values for respiratory events in overnight polygraphy from infants aged 1 and 3months. Sleep Med 2013;14(12):1323–7.
44. Vézina K, Mariasine J, Young R, et al. Cardiorespiratory Monitoring Data during Sleep in Healthy Canadian Infants. Ann Am Thorac Soc 2020;17(10):1238–46.

Adenotonsillectomy for Obstructive Sleep Apnea in Children

Samantha L. Jaensch, MBBS[a,b], Alan T. Cheng, BHB, MBCHB, FRACS[c,d], Karen A. Waters, MBBS, FRACP, PhD, GCCM[c,e,*]

KEYWORDS

• Child • Sleep-disordered breathing • OSA • Tonsillectomy • Complications

KEY POINTS

- Symptoms of obstructed breathing are the commonest indication for tonsillectomy in children.
- Polysomnography remains complex, expensive, and limited in its availability to children with symptoms of airway obstruction.
- Children with obstructive sleep apnea are at higher risk of postoperative complications than those without obstructive issues, with up to 20% experiencing respiratory compromise requiring intervention.
- Age has been demonstrated to affect the rates of post-tonsillectomy complications in several ways.
- Obesity increases the risk of post-tonsillectomy complications such as bleeding, pain, and postoperative respiratory adverse events.

INTRODUCTION

Tonsillectomy is one of the most commonly performed surgical procedures in children worldwide, with estimated 530,000 tonsillectomies with or without adenoidectomies performed in children aged less than 15 years in the United States each year.[1] Techniques and tools have changed significantly over time, and the increase in childhood

[a] Northern Clinical School, The University of Sydney, Sydney, New South Wales, Australia; [b] Sydney Medical School – Northern, L7 Kolling Building RNSH, Reserve Road, St Leonards, NSW 2065, Australia; [c] Discipline of Child and Adolescent Health, Faculty of Medicine, The University of Sydney, Sydney, New South Wales, Australia; [d] Department of Ear Nose & Throat Surgery, The Children's Hospital at Westmead, Locked Bag 4001, Westmead, NSW 2145, Australia; [e] Respiratory Support Services, The Children's Hospital at Westmead, Locked Bag 4001, Westmead, NSW 2145, Australia

* Corresponding author. SIDS and Sleep Apnoea Research, Respiratory Support Services, The Children's Hospital at Westmead, Locked Bag 4001, Westmead, NSW 2145, Australia.
E-mail address: Karen.Waters@health.nsw.gov.au

Otolaryngol Clin N Am 57 (2024) 407–419
https://doi.org/10.1016/j.otc.2024.02.025
oto.theclinics.com
0030-6665/24/

obesity as well as advancements in antibiotics over the last few decades has seen a shift in the most common indication for pediatric tonsillectomy from recurrent acute tonsillitis to obstructive sleep-disordered breathing (OSDB).[2] As a result, the goals of tonsil surgery have changed with a renewed focus on reducing unnecessary morbidity from postoperative complications.[3] This review aims to provide an overview of pediatric tonsillectomy for management of obstructive sleep apnea (OSA), to describe common post-tonsillectomy complications, and to explore risk factors for persistent OSA, including demographics, comorbidities, surgical techniques, and perioperative medications.

Terminology between methods in contemporary studies varies greatly. Terms such as *extracapsular tonsillectomy* and *total tonsillectomy* (TT) are used to describe the removal of all tonsillar tissue including the fibrous capsule from the overlying pharyngeal constrictor muscle. When a cuff of tonsillar tissue including the fibrous capsule is left, this is referred to as either *tonsillotomy*, *intracapsular tonsillectomy*, or *partial tonsillectomy* (PT). For the purposes of this review, "tonsillectomy" will be used as a general term to refer to the removal of the tonsils and where specified, "total tonsillectomy" and "partial tonsillectomy" will be used to differentiate between the two methods.

Tonsil Surgery for Obstructive Sleep Apnea

OSDB describes a spectrum of abnormalities in the pattern of respiration and oxygenation during sleep due to prolonged partial upper airway obstruction, with OSA representing the most severe cases where intermittent complete obstruction of the upper airway occurs.[4] Polysomnography (PSG) remains the gold standard for diagnosis of OSA, whereas OSDB is a clinical diagnosis based on history from caregivers.[1] An apnea–hypopnea index (AHI) greater than 1 event per hour is diagnostic of OSA, and AHI greater than 10 indicates severe OSA.[4,5]

For children with normal weight and OSDB/OSA, adenotonsillar hypertrophy is the leading cause and as such, adenotonsillectomy is recommended as first-line therapy.[4] Adenotonsillectomy has shown OSDB cure rates of up to 80% in children of normal weight[1] and while tonsil size alone does not predict the degree of obstruction, the combined volume of adenoids and tonsils does predict severity of OSDB,[6] as demonstrated by Arens and colleagues using MRI in children with and without OSA. MRI understandably is not a viable alternative to PSG for younger children due to requiring general anesthetic to tolerate. The current clinical practice guideline recommends PSG prior to tonsillectomy for children under 2 years of age or those with comorbidities such as obesity, Down syndrome, craniofacial abnormalities, or neuromuscular disorders, and also cases where the need for operative management is uncertain.[1]

Children with obesity, defined as body mass index (BMI) greater than 2 standard deviations from the mean or over 95th percentile for age and gender,[4] have twice the odds of undergoing adenotonsillectomy than healthy-weight children, according to a nationwide-wide audit of perioperative obesity in the United Kingdom by Burton and colleagues.[7] The authors identified that obese children have nearly 3 times higher rates of snoring and OSDB than overweight children, likely a combination of adenotonsillar hypertrophy and increased neck adiposity. This is in keeping with OSA rates of up to 60% in obese children compared to up to 6% of the general pediatric population.[4,8] Despite lower treatment cure rates for obese children with OSDB,[1] adenotonsillectomy remains first-line treatment according to US guidelines,[4] possibly contributing to the overrepresentation of obese children undergoing the procedure.[7]

PT began to regain popularity in the early 2000s when the technique was reintroduced to reduce oropharyngeal obstruction from the tonsils in patients with OSDB while retaining a barrier over underlying tissues as a means of preventing pain, expediting recovery, and reducing complications such as infection and bleeding.[9] A 2020 Cochrane review by Blackshaw and colleagues was unable to determine a difference in clinical effectiveness compared to TT due to the quality of available studies.[3] A drawback of PT is the possibility of tonsil regrowth and need for definitive TT. Rates of regrowth vary from 2% to 6%[10–12] and appear to be associated with younger age[12] and acute tonsillitis post-operatively.[11] Reoperation rates are generally lower (1%–2%) but revision surgery puts children at risk of general complications associated with anesthesia and surgery, as well as specific procedure-related risks.[13,14]

The addition of adenoidectomy to tonsillectomy in children is often out of necessity, either due to nasal obstruction from adenoidal hypertrophy or the combined contribution of adenotonsillar tissue to pharyngeal obstruction in OSDB.[6] However, it appears to provide some protection from risk of post-tonsillectomy hemorrhage (PTH) on multivariable models.[15] It is worth keeping in mind, however, that children undergoing adenotonsillectomy rather than tonsillectomy may be doing so for management of OSDB rather than recurrent tonsillitis, placing them at an already reduced risk of bleeding.

Day-stay, outpatient, or ambulatory tonsillectomy is commonplace in the United States with the majority of pediatric procedures being performed on an outpatient basis.[1] In Australia, a steady increase in the proportion of tonsillectomies performed as day-stay procedures has been noted over the past 2 decades from 2.7% in 2000 to 14.2% in 2020.[16] In Germany, however, inpatient tonsillectomy remains the mainstay with patients admitted for 2 to 3 days postoperatively,[17] a reduction since the early 2000s where admissions of up to 6 days were routine.[18] It is unclear whether health care-related costs influence the recommended length of stay post-tonsillectomy across countries.

Without close monitoring, some postoperative complications occurring in day-stay patients are not recorded or reported to providers, skewing the rate of complications via an observer bias. The higher rates of perioperative respiratory adverse events (PRAEs) experienced by younger children and those with OSA remain a significant concern, leading to an update in the 2019 American Clinical Guidelines recommending overnight admission for children under 3 years of age and those with AHI greater than 10 or oxygen saturation nadir less than 80%.[1] This highlights the importance of individual patient risk assessment when making the decision to perform ambulatory procedures.

Complications of Tonsil Surgery

Complications from tonsillectomy in children can be categorized by their frequency, severity, and affected system. Johnson and colleagues classified common complications by their time of onset,[19] namely primary events occurring immediately or within the first 24 hours, delayed events occurring up to 2 weeks postoperatively, and longer term complications. This review will focus on common primary and delayed complications, which include bleeding, anesthetic and respiratory issues, pain, infection, and dehydration. In Australia, the majority of children undergoing tonsillectomy will be admitted overnight for observation[16] especially where the indication for surgery is OSDB; however, this is not the case in the United States where most procedures are done in an ambulatory setting,[1] possibly reducing the visibility of primary complications.

Bleeding

By far, the most dreaded of post-tonsillectomy complications is hemorrhage. Primary PTH occurs in the first 24 hours following surgery, while secondary PTH occurs after

24 hours[20] and represents the majority of bleeding following tonsillectomy.[1] It is thought that primary PTH is a result of inadequate intraoperative hemostasis,[21] while secondary PTH occurs when necrotic slough is dislodged from the tonsillar fossae, formed as a result of thermal tissue damage during the procedure.[22] Rates vary across the literature from 1.6% to 6.7%,[23,24] with Lowe and colleagues reporting an overall 3.5% bleeding rate using the National Prospective Tonsillectomy Audit of 34,000 patients in England and Northern Ireland.[22] This is the largest primary study to date that has encompassed all events of bleeding, including those requiring a return to the operating theater and those managed conservatively.

Anesthetic and respiratory issues

The most frequent perioperative anesthetic complications of tonsillectomy include trauma and respiratory events. Laryngoscopy during intubation can cause dental trauma, temporomandibular joint dislocation, and pharyngeal soft tissue injury, while the Boyle–Davis gag—used to provide visualization to the oropharynx during tonsillectomy—can contribute to the same injuries as well as accidental extubation and impaired ventilation by compression of the endotracheal tube.[19] PRAEs may occur such as upper airway obstruction, post-obstructive pulmonary edema, and hypoxemia,[25,26] and these may require interventions ranging from supplemental oxygen to reintubation and ventilatory support.[27]

Postoperative infection

Lower respiratory tract infections can occur due to aspiration of blood or secretions or atelectasis from decreased alveolar recruitment.[28] Surgical edema may cause eustachian tube dysfunction, particularly when adenoidectomy is performed, and this can cause a secondary otitis media, either acute or with effusion.[1] Surgical-site infection following tonsillectomy is rare but remains a common misdiagnosis due to the sloughy appearance of the tonsillar fossae during the first 2 weeks of recovery.

Pain

Effective management of postoperative pain is imperative in patients recovering from tonsillectomy, as consequences of pain in this region include limited oral intake, dehydration, sleep disturbance, behavioral changes, and hospital readmission.[29] Identification of pain in pediatric patients can be challenging for caregivers due to communication barriers and emotional distress, and several pain rating scales such as the Wong-Baker FACES scale and the face, legs, activity, cry, consolability (FLACC) pain scale have been developed and validated.[30,31] Pain management is further complicated by parental concerns, misunderstanding regarding analgesia, and children's refusal of oral medications.[1] Many patients recovering from tonsillectomy not only experience immediate postoperative pain, but also a delayed worsening of pain often around postoperative days 5 to 7 referred to in the literature as the pain peak or postoperative dip,[32] the exact cause of which is not well understood.

Dehydration

It is crucial that children recovering from tonsillectomy are able to manage adequate oral intake, facilitated by effective analgesia, to prevent dehydration and need for readmission.[33] Dehydration can also lead to increased pain, developing a vicious cycle when children are unable to manage oral intake due to oropharyngeal pain. Hypovolemia, whether due to blood loss or decreased oral intake, can be particularly severe in children due to reduced circulating volume[34] and vital signs are a poor marker in children for the severity of volume deficit.

RISK FACTORS FOR COMPLICATIONS

Patient Factors

Obstructive sleep apnea versus other indications

Children with OSA are at higher risk of postoperative complications than those without obstructive issues, with up to 20% experiencing respiratory compromise requiring intervention.[35] Despite removal of the presumed cause of obstruction, children with OSA have still been shown to experience higher rates of PRAEs following adenotonsillectomy,[26,36] with a meta-analysis by De Luca Canto and colleagues identifying an overall odds ratio (OR) for post-tonsillectomy respiratory complications of 4.90 compared to children without OSA.[37] Nixon and colleagues demonstrated marked sleep disturbance, desaturations, and obstructive events on PSGs performed on the first night following adenotonsillectomy for OSA. Those with mild OSA (AHI between 1 and 5 on preoperative PSG) had an average AHI of 6.9 on postoperative PSG the first-night post-adenotonsillectomy, and for children with severe OSA, the average AHI was 21.5.[38] They noted that there was no significant difference in perioperative medications or volume of adenotonsillar tissue removed between the mild and severe groups. Interestingly, the child with the most severe obstructive events postoperatively in the Nixon study went on to have normal nocturnal oximetry 6 weeks later.[38]

Some predictors of post-tonsillectomy PRAEs for children with OSA have been identified in the literature. Billings and colleagues demonstrated that children with PSG showing AHI greater than 27 events per hour, greater than 18.5 obstructive apneas, and an oxygen saturation nadir of less than 72% were at higher risk of postoperative respiratory events requiring interventions such as supplementary oxygen and reintubation.[5] Xiao and colleagues found that the McGill oximetry score on PSG was a more accurate parameter in predicting PRAEs than AHI following adenotonsillectomy,[25] suggesting that simple nocturnal oximetry can provide most of the essential information needed for post-tonsillectomy monitoring. This strengthens the recommendation that children with severe OSA be admitted for continuous oxygen saturation monitoring following adenotonsillectomy.

Much of the literature on post-tonsillectomy complications experienced by children with OSA is regarding respiratory events, with far fewer studies focusing on other complications. De Luca Canto demonstrated in their meta-analysis that children with OSA were less likely to experience PTH than those without, calculating an OR of 0.41 for this group.[37] Gerhke and colleagues calculated a secondary PTH rate for children with OSA of 1.9% compared to 0.8% for non-OSA[36]; however, only complications within the first 24 hours were included, reducing the likelihood of capturing bleeding events and the raising questions regarding the classification of secondary bleeding in their study. Achar and colleagues analyzed a group of pediatric patients presenting with post-tonsillectomy complications and found an increased risk of PTH in those operated on for OSA compared to tonsillitis. However, different data sources were used to identify the number of tonsillectomies performed and the number of PTH presentations in the study timeframe.[39]

Demographics

Age has been demonstrated to affect the rates of post-tonsillectomy complications in several ways. Younger children experience up to 3 time higher rates of total postoperative complications, especially PRAEs[40] and events occurring in the first 24 hours.[41] Interestingly, the risk of post-tonsillectomy bleeding increases with age,[42,43] with a national US study showing that children between 5 and 11 years of age and those over 12 years old were 1.5 and 3 times more likely to experience a bleed than those less than 5 year old.[23] It is well established that male patients will experience higher rates of bleeding up to 1.8 times those of their female counterparts,[16,21,23,44,45] despite the underlying reasons being poorly understood. Gender has not been shown to significantly affect rates of other post-tonsillectomy complications. Caucasian ethnicity appears to be associated with lower rates of readmission following tonsillectomy[44,46,47]; however, no studies have demonstrated an association between race or ethnicity and PTH. Lower socioeconomic status appears to increase risk of all post-tonsillectomy complications.[44,47]

Comorbidities

Obesity increases the risk of post-tonsillectomy complications such as bleeding, pain, and PRAEs. Children with BMI greater than 85th percentile have over twice the odds of PTH[48–50] and over twice the duration of pain than children with normal weight.[51] Children with obesity experience increased rates of intraoperative desaturation, multiple laryngoscopy attempts, difficult mask ventilation, postoperative airway obstruction, longer lengths of stay[52] and show similar obstructive and hypoxic parameters on PSG performed the night of tonsillectomy as their preoperative studies.[8] The presence of complex chronic conditions including Down syndrome and prematurity puts children at nearly double the risk of readmission for dehydration and pain.[33,46] In medically complex children, identified predictors of PRAEs include craniofacial conditions (OR 4.97), cardiac abnormalities (OR 2.07–2.09), airway anomalies (OR 3.19–3.48), neurologic conditions (OR 2.36), genetic disorders (OR 2.04), and a history of prematurity (OR 6.23).[27,53] Down syndrome confers a higher risk of OSA, but following tonsillectomy has a morbidity rate of up to 31.5% and a PTH rate of 17.9%.[54] It is estimated that only 30% to 40% of children with Down syndrome will have resolution of OSA symptoms after adenotonsillectomy,[4] with some even demonstrating worsening OSA on postoperative PSG.[55] Asthma increases the likelihood of readmission for pain and dehydration[46] but was not identified as a predictor for PRAEs following tonsillectomy. Reflux disorders increase risk of PRAEs including aspiration pneumonitis, hypoxemia and the need for reintubation,[56] delayed pain, PTH, and longer postoperative stay.[57] Attention deficit hyperactivity disorder (ADHD) was identified as a significant risk factor for PTH with a relative risk of 8.7[43]; however, multivariate analyses in other studies have shown a decreased risk, suggesting that other factors were likely to be contributing to bleeding risk.[49] ADHD is associated with increased readmission for pain and dehydration.[46]

Perioperative Factors

Methods of dissection and hemostasis

"Cold" methods of tonsillectomy utilize sharp steel instruments for dissection, and ligatures or ties for hemostasis, while "hot" methods use electrocautery devices or other similarly powered instruments for dissection and hemostasis. These include monopolar diathermy wands, bipolar scissors, bipolar forceps, coblation, and less commonly, laser, harmonic scalpel, and radiofrequency ablation. Several large retrospective studies have reported increased rates of primary PTH with all hot methods when compared to cold dissection,[21,22] with some even reporting higher likelihood of PTH if cold dissection is accompanied with bipolar hemostasis rather than ties.[58] Despite multiple studies demonstrating lower secondary PTH risk with cold methods, the increased intraoperative blood loss and higher rates of primary PTH are considered hard to rationalize in pediatric patients.[59] Cautery methods were associated with increased readmission rates for pain and dehydration when compared to cold dissection and coblation tonsillectomies.[46]

Total versus partial tonsillectomy

By preventing exposure and injury to the pharyngeal constrictor muscles, PT appears to improve pain outcomes for children postoperatively, with several systematic reviews demonstrating shorter duration of pain, fewer doses of analgesia, and a quicker return to normal diet compared to TT.[60–62] In studies comparing coblation TT to coblation PT, there was no difference in severity of early pain but PT appeared to prevent the postoperative dip[32] and showed significantly lower rates of secondary PTH.[60]

In a Swedish national patient registry cohort study, Odhagen and colleagues demonstrated that the risk of postoperative complications from completion tonsillectomy following PT was greater than that of TT performed as a primary procedure, with a PTH rate of 4% for secondary completion versus 2.5% for primary TT.[15] Bagwell and colleagues studied the cost-effectiveness of PT and concluded that until the rate of regrowth requiring completion tonsillectomy remained consistently less than 3.1%, TT would remain the most cost-effective option for management of childhood OSA despite its increased rates of readmission.[63]

Choice of analgesia

Post-tonsillectomy pain management for children with OSDB remains an area of controversy. Paracetamol or acetaminophen remains the first-line treatment, with nonsteroidal anti-inflammatory drugs (NSAIDs) being second line. However, despite a large body of evidence including multiple Cochrane reviews, concerns regarding the risk of PTH with NSAIDs persist.[1] Ibuprofen is a nonselective cyclooxygenase (COX) inhibitor with demonstrated effects on platelet aggregation posing a theoretically increased risk of bleeding, and a 2013 Cochrane review by Lewis and colleagues concluded that there was insufficient evidence to exclude an increased risk of bleeding.[64] Celecoxib is an oral selective COX-2 inhibitor that does not have the same impact on platelet aggregation and has demonstrated lower rates of PTH compared to ibuprofen, but is not recommended for children under the age of 12 years.[42] Parecoxib is a long-acting COX-2 inhibitor that can be given as a single intravenous dose on induction of general anesthesia for tonsillectomy, with evidence to suggest significantly reduced early postoperative pain, opioid requirement, and postoperative nausea and vomiting,[65] and no increase in the risk of primary or secondary PTH.[66] In 2013, the US Food and Drug Administration identified 10 children under the age of 9 years who had died from respiratory depression following administration of weight-appropriate doses of codeine post-tonsillectomy,[1] the majority of which were found to be ultrarapid metabolizers of codeine to morphine that in combination with a diagnosis of OSA would have significantly increased their risk of respiratory depression.[1,53] Alternative opioid agents such as oxycodone have been shown to produce effective pain relief with less sedation[67] but can still increase the risk of PRAEs, nausea, vomiting, and constipation in children post-tonsillectomy.[64,68] Local anesthetic agents such as lidocaine, bupivacaine, and ropivacaine given as intraoperative injections either before or after tonsillar dissection have been demonstrated to produce less severe pain, reduced analgesia requirements including opioid analgesia, and no difference in complications compared to placebo.[30,69]

CONTROVERSIES IN THE TWENTY-FIRST CENTURY

PSG remains complex, expensive, and limited in its availability to children with symptoms of airway obstruction. The European Respiratory Society Task Force recognizes that PSG may not be available to all children but states that no currently available alternative methods can substitute for PSG.[70] In the absence of any other reliable and readily available diagnostic test for OSA, many children therefore undergo surgery on the basis of their clinical history and physical findings alone. In a recent review of 1409 children who underwent tonsillectomy at our hospital, eradication of symptoms was 44% higher following tonsillectomy in children without a preoperative sleep study compared to those with a diagnosis of OSA on sleep study. For children who had PSG before surgery, in the 5 years following their surgery less than 4% had a follow-up PSG to document the success, or not, of their surgery.

Regarding outcomes of tonsillectomy for OSA assessed using PSG criteria, 3 large, randomized studies have been undertaken in children. The Childhood Adenotonsillectomy Trial study randomized 464 children, aged 5 to 9 years, to tonsillectomy or watchful waiting with follow-up after 7 months.[71] The Pre-school OSA Tonsillectomy Adenoidectomy study randomized 190 preschool children, aged 3 to 5 years with mild-to-moderate OSA on PSG, to early (within 2 months) or delayed adenotonsillectomy with follow-up at 12 months and then at 24 months after all children had undergone surgery. Both studies included neurocognition as the primary outcome and found modest, if any changes in cognitive outcomes. However, secondary analyses of the outcomes have demonstrated that children who underwent surgery had improvements in symptom burden, sleepiness (on questionnaire and by reduction in daytime napping in the preschool age-group), parent-reported behavior, and quality of life.[72,73] The most recent study examined outcomes of early adenotonsillectomy compared to supportive care in 459 children aged 3 to 12.9 years, with an obstructive AHI of less than 3 per hour, and therefore deemed to have only mild disease, to early adenotonsillectomy or watchful waiting and followed up at 12 months.[74] Again, it was found that sleepiness, behavioral problems, and quality of life improved more with adenotonsillectomy that with medical care, and that with blood pressure (as a measure of cardiovascular function) also improved. But the association between the PSG measures and the various outcomes was limited.[72]

In studies where PSG was used to evaluate the severity of OSA, tonsillectomy was demonstrated to improve sleep, daytime behaviour and blood pressure even in very mild cases of OSA.[73–75] Insistence by governments or insurers that children have a positive diagnosis of OSA on PSG before surgery raises the question of whether a significant population of children who stand to benefit from tonsillectomy may be denied the procedure even if they have PSG with an apnea index below accepted thresholds. Linked to this is the question of whether the PSG measurements, and certainly the outcome of the AHI, accurately reflect the pathology of airway obstruction in these children. Physiologic studies and tools using other measurements have demonstrated that periods of partial obstruction and the changes that occur postoperatively in a child's breathing are not accurately represented by the apnea index of PSG.[76,77] Ongoing research is still required to identify appropriate measurement tools to guide indications and outcomes of surgery.

SUMMARY

Although much research has been done on risk factors for complications of pediatric tonsillectomy in terms of patient factors such as demographics and comorbidities as well as procedure-related factors such as technique, instruments, and perioperative medications, yet there are many areas where the evidence remains conflicted. Current areas of controversy include which method of tonsillectomy confers the greatest advantage to particular patient groups and whether ibuprofen has a clinically meaningful effect on PTH. The latter issue may see some clarification if rates of ibuprofen administration continue to rise in response to the 2019 guidelines. However, the literature does agree on several points, namely that male gender and increasing age are associated with increased risk of PTH, recurrent tonsillitis as an indication for surgery may result in more pain and higher rates of PTH, and that while cold steel tonsillectomy contributes to less secondary PTH than cautery methods, the increased intraoperative blood loss in children cannot be ignored. While further high-quality studies need to be performed to definitively answer remaining questions, ENT surgeons and other health care providers need to be able to draw their own conclusions from the available evidence in terms of what methods will achieve optimal results for their patients. As a mentor once said to me, "the best method is the one that is safest in my hands."

CLINICS CARE POINTS

- Tonsillectomy is the commonest ENT surgery performed on paediatric patients in the USA, with oSDB (including OSA) the leading indication for surgery in this group - yet children with OSA experience higher rates of post-tonsillectomy complications especially PRAEs.
- OSA rates are increasing worldwide, in part due to increasing rates of childhood obesity which in itself increases the risk of PTH, PRAEs and pain following tonsillectomy.
- Children may demonstrate a similar or even worse degree of obstruction on the first night post-tonsillectomy despite the presumed source of obstruction being removed, which reiterates the importance of overnight monitoring for children with severe OSA on pre-operative PSG.
- The severity of OSA does not always predict the degree of improvement in obstruction post-tonsillectomy, and children with very mild pre-operative disease on PSG can have significant improvements in sleep quality, daytime behaviour and blood pressure following tonsillectomy.
- While PSG remains the gold standard for OSA diagnosis, a more affordable and accessible measure of the impact of the disease needs to be developed to ensure that children who stand to benefit from tonsillectomy are not denied the procedure based on availability and severity of PSG results.

REFERENCES

1. Mitchell RB, Archer SM, Ishman SL, et al. Clinical practice guideline: tonsillectomy in children (update). Otolaryngol Head Neck Surg 2019;160(1_suppl):S1–42.
2. Parker NP, Walner DL. Trends in the indications for pediatric tonsillectomy or adenotonsillectomy. Int J Pediatr Otorhinolaryngol 2011;75(2):282–5.
3. Blackshaw H, Springford LR, Zhang LY, et al. Tonsillectomy versus tonsillotomy for obstructive sleep-disordered breathing in children. Cochrane Database Syst Rev 2020;4(4):CD011365.
4. Marcus CL, Brooks LJ, Draper KA, et al. Diagnosis and management of childhood obstructive sleep apnea syndrome. Pediatrics 2012;130(3):576–84.
5. Billings KR, Somani SN, Lavin J, et al. Polysomnography variables associated with postoperative respiratory issues in children <3 Years of age undergoing adenotonsillectomy for obstructive sleep apnea. Int J Pediatr Otorhinolaryngol 2020;137:110215.
6. Arens R, McDonough JM, Corbin AM, et al. Upper airway size analysis by magnetic resonance imaging of children with obstructive sleep apnea syndrome. Am J Respir Crit Care Med 2003;167(1):65–70.
7. Burton ZA, Lewis R, Bennett T, et al. Prevalence of PErioperAtive CHildhood obesitY in children undergoing general anaesthesia in the UK: a prospective, multicentre, observational cohort study. Br J Anaesth 2021;127(6):953–61.

8. De A, Waltuch T, Gonik NJ, et al. Sleep and breathing the first night after adenotonsillectomy in obese children with obstructive sleep apnea. J Clin Sleep Med 2017;13(6):805–11.
9. Koltai PJ, Solares CA, Koempel JA, et al. Intracapsular tonsillar reduction (partial tonsillectomy): reviving a historical procedure for obstructive sleep disordered breathing in children. Otolaryngol Head Neck Surg 2003;129(5):532–8.
10. Chang D, Zemek A, Koltai P. Comparison of treatment outcomes between intracapsular and total tonsillectomy for pediatric obstructive sleep apnea. Int J Pediatr Otorhinolaryngol 2016;91. https://doi.org/10.1016/j.ijporl.2016.09.029.
11. Zhang Q, Li D, Wang H. Long term outcome of tonsillar regrowth after partial tonsillectomy in children with obstructive sleep apnea. Auris Nasus Larynx 2014; 41(3):299–302.
12. Tipirneni KE, Bauter L, Sher ET, et al. Identifying cohort differences in children undergoing partial intracapsular tonsillectomy vs traditional tonsillectomy for sleep disordered breathing. Int J Pediatr Otorhinolaryngol 2020;137:110183.
13. Sagheer SH, Kolb CM, Crippen MM, et al. Predictive pediatric characteristics for revision tonsillectomy after intracapsular tonsillectomy. Otolaryngol Head Neck Surg 2022;166(4):772–8.
14. Sathe N, Chinnadurai S, McPheeters M, et al. Comparative effectiveness of partial versus total tonsillectomy in children. Otolaryngol Head Neck Surg 2017; 156(3):456–63.
15. Odhagen E, Stalfors J, Sunnergren O. Morbidity after pediatric tonsillotomy versus tonsillectomy: A population-based cohort study. Laryngoscope 2019; 129(11):2619–26.
16. Li JC, Forer M, Veivers D. Reference rate for post-tonsillectomy haemorrhage in Australia-A 2000-2020 national hospital morbidity database analysis. PLoS One 2022;17(8):e0273320.
17. Mueller J, Boeger D, Buentzel J, et al. Population-based analysis of tonsil surgery and postoperative hemorrhage. Eur Arch Oto-Rhino-Laryngol 2015;272(12): 3769–77.
18. Schrock A, Send T, Heukamp L, et al. The role of histology and other risk factors for post-tonsillectomy haemorrhage. Eur Arch Oto-Rhino-Laryngol 2009;266(12): 1983–7.
19. Johnson LB, Elluru RG, Myer CM 3rd. Complications of adenotonsillectomy. Laryngoscope 2002;112(8 Pt 2 Suppl 100):35–6.
20. Windfuhr JP, Chen YS, Remmert S. Hemorrhage following tonsillectomy and adenoidectomy in 15,218 patients. Otolaryngol Head Neck Surg 2005;132(2): 281–6.
21. Tomkinson A, Harrison W, Owens D, et al. Risk factors for postoperative hemorrhage following tonsillectomy. Laryngoscope 2011;121(2):279–88.
22. Lowe D, van der Meulen J, Cromwell D, et al. Key messages from the national prospective tonsillectomy audit. Laryngoscope 2007;117(4):717–24.
23. Leung P, DeVore EK, Kawai K, et al. Does ibuprofen increase bleed risk for pediatric tonsillectomy? Otolaryngology-Head Neck Surg (Tokyo) 2021;165(1): 187–96.
24. Granell J, Gete P, Villafruela M, et al. Safety of outpatient tonsillectomy in children: a review of 6 years in a tertiary hospital experience. Otolaryngol Head Neck Surg 2004;131(4):383–7.
25. Xiao L, Barrowman N, Momoli F, et al. Polysomnography parameters as predictors of respiratory adverse events following adenotonsillectomy in children. J Clin Sleep Med 2021;17(11):2215–23.

26. Kieran S, Gorman C, Kirby A, et al. Risk factors for desaturation after tonsillectomy: analysis of 4092 consecutive pediatric cases. Laryngoscope 2013;123(10):2554–9.
27. Katz SL, Monsour A, Barrowman N, et al. Predictors of postoperative respiratory complications in children undergoing adenotonsillectomy. J Clin Sleep Med 2020;16(1):41–8.
28. Rasmussen N. Complications of tonsillectomy and adenoidectomy. Otolaryngol Clin North Am 1987;20(2):383–90.
29. Curtis JL, Harvey DB, Willie S, et al. Causes and costs for ED visits after pediatric adenotonsillectomy. Otolaryngol Head Neck Surg 2015;152(4):691–6.
30. Stramiello JA, Ortega B, Brigger M, et al. Effect of local anesthetic injections on subjective pain scales in pediatric tonsillectomies: a meta-analysis. Otolaryngol Head Neck Surg 2022. https://doi.org/10.1177/01945998221094228. 1945998221094228.
31. Redmann AJ, Wang Y, Furstein J, et al. The use of the FLACC pain scale in pediatric patients undergoing adenotonsillectomy. Int J Pediatr Otorhinolaryngol 2017;92:115–8.
32. Daskalakis D, Tsetsos N, Karagergou S, et al. Intracapsular coblation tonsillectomy versus extracapsular coblation tonsillectomy: a systematic review and a meta-analysis. Eur Arch Oto-Rhino-Laryngol 2021;278(3):637–44.
33. Hession-Laband E, Melvin P, Shermont H, et al. Reducing readmissions post-tonsillectomy: a quality improvement study on intravenous hydration. J Healthc Qual 2018;40(4):217–27.
34. Wood JM, Harris PK, Woods CM, et al. Quality of life following surgery for sleep disordered breathing: subtotal reduction adenotonsillectomy versus adenotonsillectomy in Australian children. ANZ J Surg 2011;81(5):340–4.
35. Rosen GM, Muckle RP, Mahowald MW, et al. Postoperative respiratory compromise in children with obstructive sleep apnea syndrome: can it be anticipated? Pediatrics 1994;93(5):784–8.
36. Gehrke T, Scherzad A, Hagen R, et al. Risk factors for children requiring adenotonsillectomy and their impact on postoperative complications: a retrospective analysis of 2000 patients. Anaesthesia 2019;74(12):1572–9.
37. De Luca Canto G, Pacheco-Pereira C, Aydinoz S, et al. Adenotonsillectomy complications: a meta-analysis. Pediatrics 2015;136(4):702–18.
38. Nixon GM, Kermack AS, McGregor CD, et al. Sleep and breathing on the first night after adenotonsillectomy for obstructive sleep apnea. Pediatr Pulmonol 2005;39(4):332–8.
39. Achar P, Sharma RK, De S, et al. Does primary indication for tonsillectomy influence post-tonsillectomy haemorrhage rates in children? Int J Pediatr Otorhinolaryngol 2015;79(2):246–50.
40. Cooper F, Spektor Z, Kay DJ. Rate and risk factors for post-adenotonsillectomy complications in children under 24 months and 24 to 36 months old. Am J Otolaryngol 2020;41(4):102546.
41. Lawlor C, Riley C, Carter J, et al. Association between age and weight as risk factors for complication after tonsillectomy in healthy children. JAMA Otolaryngology - Head and Neck Surgery 2018;144. https://doi.org/10.1001/jamaoto.2017.3431.
42. Kwok MW, Subramaniyan M, Rimmer J, et al. Post-tonsillectomy haemorrhage in Australia - a multivariable analysis of risk factors. review. Aust J Oto Laryngol 2018;1(1):2.
43. Spektor Z, Saint-Victor S, Kay DJ, et al. Risk factors for pediatric post-tonsillectomy hemorrhage. Int J Pediatr Otorhinolaryngol 2016;84:151–5.

44. Bhattacharyya N, Shapiro NL. Associations between socioeconomic status and race with complications after tonsillectomy in children. Otolaryngol Head Neck Surg 2014;151(6):1055–60.
45. Harju T, Numminen J. Risk factors for secondary post-tonsillectomy haemorrhage following tonsillectomy with bipolar scissors: Four-year retrospective cohort study. J Laryngol Otol 2016;131:1–7.
46. Lavin J, Lehmann D, Silva AL, et al. Variables associated with pediatric emergency department visits for uncontrolled pain in postoperative adenotonsillectomy patients. Int J Pediatr Otorhinolaryngol 2019;123:10–4.
47. Lloyd AM, Behzadpour HK, Schonman I, et al. Socioeconomic factors associated with readmission following pediatric tonsillectomy. Int J Pediatr Otorhinolaryngol 2021;151:110917.
48. Johnston J, Vergeer A, Donaldson N, et al. Our experience of the increased rates of post tonsillectomy haemorrhage in 1538 children with pre-operative infective symptoms or signs. Clin Otolaryngol 2020;45. https://doi.org/10.1111/coa.13610.
49. Kolb C, Jain N, Schillinger K, et al. Does perioperative ketorolac increase bleeding risk after intracapsular tonsillectomy? Int J Pediatr Otorhinolaryngol 2021;147:110781.
50. McKeon M, Kirsh E, Kawai K, et al. Risk factors for multiple hemorrhages following tonsil surgery in children. Laryngoscope 2019;129(12):2765–70.
51. Martin SD, John LD. Implications of a retrospective study on weight-based risk for post-tonsillectomy pain in children. J Perianesth Nurs 2020;35(2):140–6.
52. Nafiu OO, Green GE, Walton S, et al. Obesity and risk of peri-operative complications in children presenting for adenotonsillectomy. Int J Pediatr Otorhinolaryngol 2009;73(1):89–95.
53. Tsampalieros A, Murto K, Barrowman N, et al. Opioid dose and postoperative respiratory adverse events after adenotonsillectomy in medically complex children. J Clin Sleep Med 2022;18(10):2405–13.
54. Cottrell J, Zahr SK, Propst EJ, et al. Morbidity and mortality from adenotonsillectomy in children with trisomy 21. Int J Pediatr Otorhinolaryngol 2020;138:110377.
55. Abijay CA, Tomkies A, Rayasam S, et al. Children with down syndrome and obstructive sleep apnea: outcomes after tonsillectomy. Otolaryngol Head Neck Surg 2022;166(3):557–64.
56. Chorney S, Zur K, Buzi A. Reflux as a risk factor for morbidity after pediatric tonsillectomy: a national cohort of inpatients. Laryngoscope 2020;131. https://doi.org/10.1002/lary.28895.
57. Salturk Z, Kumral TL, Arslanoglu A, et al. Role of laryngopharyngeal reflux in complications of tonsillectomy in pediatric patients. Indian J Otolaryngol Head Neck Surg 2017;69(3):392–6.
58. Sarny S, Ossimitz G, Habermann W, et al. Hemorrhage following tonsil surgery: a multicenter prospective study. Laryngoscope 2011;121(12):2553–60.
59. Shotts SD, Welsh DV, Nakamura A, et al. Very-low energy monopolar reduces post-tonsillectomy hemorrhage versus standard energy techniques. Laryngoscope 2021;131(11):2505–11.
60. Walton J, Ebner Y, Stewart MG, et al. Systematic review of randomized controlled trials comparing intracapsular tonsillectomy with total tonsillectomy in a pediatric population. Arch Otolaryngol Head Neck Surg 2012;138(3):243–9.
61. Acevedo JL, Shah RK, Brietzke SE. Systematic review of complications of tonsillotomy versus tonsillectomy. Otolaryngol Head Neck Surg 2012;146(6):871–9.

62. Zhang LY, Zhong L, David M, et al. Tonsillectomy or tonsillotomy? A systematic review for paediatric sleep-disordered breathing. Int J Pediatr Otorhinolaryngol 2017;103:41–50.
63. Bagwell K, Wu X, Baum ED, et al. Cost-effectiveness analysis of intracapsular tonsillectomy and total tonsillectomy for pediatric obstructive sleep apnea. Appl Health Econ Health Policy 2018;16(4):527–35.
64. Lewis SR, Nicholson A, Cardwell ME, et al. Nonsteroidal anti-inflammatory drugs and perioperative bleeding in paediatric tonsillectomy. Cochrane Database Syst Rev 2013;2013(7):CD003591.
65. Li X, Zhou M, Xia Q, et al. Parecoxib sodium reduces the need for opioids after tonsillectomy in children: a double-blind placebo-controlled randomized clinical trial. Can J Anaesth 2016;63(3):268–74.
66. Tan L, Taylor E, Hannam JA, et al. Pharmacokinetics and analgesic effectiveness of intravenous parecoxib for tonsillectomy +/- adenoidectomy. Paediatr Anaesth 2016;26(12):1126–35.
67. Tan GX, Tunkel DE. Control of pain after tonsillectomy in children: a review. JAMA Otolaryngol Head Neck Surg 2017;143(9):937–42.
68. Chua KP, Harbaugh CM, Brummett CM, et al. Association of perioperative opioid prescriptions with risk of complications after tonsillectomy in children. JAMA Otolaryngol Head Neck Surg 2019;145(10):911–8.
69. Sun J, Wu X, Meng Y, et al. Bupivacaine versus normal saline for relief of post-adenotonsillectomy pain in children: a meta-analysis. Int J Pediatr Otorhinolaryngol 2010;74(4):369–73.
70. Kaditis AG, Alonso Alvarez ML, Boudewyns A, et al. Obstructive sleep disordered breathing in 2- to 18-year-old children: diagnosis and management. Eur Respir J 2016;47(1):69–94.
71. Marcus CL, Moore RH, Rosen CL, et al. A randomized trial of adenotonsillectomy for childhood sleep apnea. N Engl J Med 2013;368(25):2366–76.
72. Decuzzi J, Redline S, Isaiah A. Secondary analyses of the childhood adenotonsillectomy trial: a narrative review. JAMA Otolaryngol Head Neck Surg 2022;148(8):779–84.
73. Waters KA, Chawla J, Harris MA, et al. Cognition after early tonsillectomy for mild OSA. Pediatrics 2020;145(2). https://doi.org/10.1542/peds.2019-1450.
74. Redline S, Cook K, Chervin RD, et al. Adenotonsillectomy for snoring and mild sleep apnea in children: a randomized clinical trial. JAMA 2023;330(21):2084–95.
75. Mitchell RB, Cook K, Garetz S, et al. Clinical characteristics of primary snoring vs mild obstructive sleep apnea in children: analysis of the pediatric adenotonsillectomy for snoring (PATS) randomized clinical trial. JAMA Otolaryngol Head Neck Surg 2023. https://doi.org/10.1001/jamaoto.2023.3816.
76. Norman MB, Middleton S, Erskine O, et al. Validation of the Sonomat: a contactless monitoring system used for the diagnosis of sleep disordered breathing. Sleep 2014;37(9):1477–87.
77. Norman MB, Harrison HC, Sullivan CE, et al. Measurement of snoring and stertor using the Sonomat to assess effectiveness of upper airway surgery in children. J Clin Sleep Med 2022;18(6):1649–56.

Surgical Management of Pediatric Obstructive Sleep Apnea Beyond Adenotonsillectomy

The Nose, Nasopharynx, and Palate

Nicholas R. Lenze, MD, MPH[a], Suhas R. Bharadwaj, MD[b], Christina M. Baldassari, MD[b], Erin M. Kirkham, MD, MPH[a,*]

KEYWORDS

• Obstructive sleep apnea • Pediatric • Septoplasty • Adenoidectomy • Palate • Turbinates • Nasal

KEY POINTS

- Patients with persistent obstructive sleep apnea (OSA) after adenotonsillectomy should be evaluated for additional sites of obstruction which may include the inferior turbinates, nasal septum, nasopharynx (adenoid regrowth), and palate.
- Drug-induced sleep endoscopy is helpful for identifying additional sites of obstruction in persistent pediatric OSA after adenotonsillectomy and can also be used up-front for pediatric patients with severe OSA or small tonsils on clinical examination.
- Some targeted surgical options for pediatric OSA include: submucous inferior turbinate resection, septoplasty, adenoidectomy, and expansion sphincter pharyngoplasty.

INTRODUCTION/HISTORY/DEFINITIONS/BACKGROUND

Several studies have demonstrated an association between nasal pathology and pediatric obstructive sleep apnea (OSA).[1–5] Nasal obstruction symptoms are common in children with OSA, and children with OSA are at increased risk for allergic rhinitis compared to their nonsnoring peers.[6–8] Researchers have postulated that the Starling

Funding sources: Dr E.M. Kirkham is supported by NIH NHLBI (1K23HL153897); C.M. Baldassari is supported by the following NIH Grants: 1R61HL165366-01, 5U01DC019279-03, 1R61HL165345-01.
[a] Department of Otolaryngology–Head & Neck Surgery, The University of Michigan, University of Michigan Medical Center, 1500 East Medical Center Drive, Ann Arbor, MI 48109, USA; [b] Department of Otolaryngology–Head and Neck Surgery, Eastern Virginia Medical School, 600 Gresham Drive, Suite 1100, Norfolk, VA 23507, USA
* Corresponding author. University of Michigan Medical Center, 1540 East Hospital Drive CW 5-702, SPC 4241, Ann Arbor, MI 48109.
E-mail address: ekirkham@umich.edu

Otolaryngol Clin N Am 57 (2024) 421–430
https://doi.org/10.1016/j.otc.2024.02.008 oto.theclinics.com

resistor model of airway obstruction may play a role in this association. This model assumes the airway is like a hollow tube with a collapsible segment (the pharynx). Thus, when the nasal airway is obstructed, the high resistance increases intraluminal pressure that leads to pharyngeal collapse and may worsen airway obstruction.

The most common causes of nasal obstruction in children include rhinitis, adenoid hypertrophy, turbinate hypertrophy, and septal deviation. While medical management with topical nasal steroids and antihistamines is typically first-line treatment, surgical intervention may be necessary due to persistent symptoms or difficulty with medication compliance.

While nasal surgery does not improve polysomnography (PSG) parameters in adult patients with nasal pathology, nasal surgery can improve quality of life (QOL) and sleep quality.[9,10] Likewise, early evidence suggests that surgery to relieve nasal obstruction in children may improve OSA treatment outcomes.[3] While adenotonsillectomy is the primary treatment of OSA in children, 25% to 60% of children will have persistent OSA after surgery.[11] Persistent OSA is defined as an apnea–hypopnea index (AHI) greater than 1 event per hour on PSG with symptoms or an AHI greater than 5 events per hour without symptoms after tonsillectomy with or without adenoidectomy.[11] Risk factors for persistent OSA include obesity, older age (>7 years), black race, severe preoperative OSA, trisomy 21, neuromuscular disorders, and craniofacial abnormalities.[12]

Studies of drug-induced sleep endoscopy (DISE) for pediatric OSA have found that the nose and palate are common sites of obstruction beyond the tonsils and adenoids.[2,11] While a single scoring system for pediatric DISE has yet to be universally adopted, a recently proposed consensus scoring rubric includes an assessment of the nasal cavity, nasopharynx, and the palate among the sites scored.[13] Common indications for pediatric DISE include small tonsils, severe baseline OSA, and persistent post-adenotonsillectomy OSA.[2] A consensus statement panel agreed that children who undergo DISE-directed surgery do experience improved surgical outcomes in terms of both PSG parameters and QOL.[2] However, prospective research is needed to assess whether surgery to improve nasal and palate obstruction results in improved pediatric OSA outcomes.

Clinical assessment of persistent snoring and both daytime and nighttime nasal airway obstruction can also be helpful for decision making. Examination with awake endoscopy in clinic is useful for identification of turbinate hypertrophy, septal deviation, and adenoid regrowth. In cases where this is not tolerated, lateral plain films can identify enlarged adenoids. This study highlights surgical management of the nose, nasopharynx, and palate in children. Procedures directed at these sites of obstruction can be performed in conjunction with adenotonsillectomy or reserved for cases of persistent OSA.

DISCUSSION

Inferior Turbinate

The nasal turbinate is responsible for warming and humidifying air as it passes from the nasal cavity to the nasopharynx. The inferior turbinate hypertrophy is responsible for a significant proportion of nasal resistance.[14] Inferior turbinates are typically assessed clinically by anterior rhinoscopy; however, there is no widely accepted definition or validated scoring system for pediatric turbinate hypertrophy. The diagnosis of turbinate hypertrophy depends both upon the degree of obstruction appreciated on examination as well as child and caregiver reports of obstructive symptoms.

Turbinate surgery has become a more common treatment approach in children with nasal obstruction and turbinate hypertrophy.[15] The increase in pediatric turbinate surgery is due, in part, to advances in device technology as well as published data that have demonstrated both safety and efficacy.[8] Two of the most common surgical techniques utilized to treat children with nasal obstruction and turbinate hypertrophy are submucosal inferior turbinate resection (SITR) and inferior turbinate cautery.[8,9] Limited data suggest that these techniques are equally efficacious for improvement of nasal obstructive symptoms in children. For the cautery technique, a turbinate cautery wand is typically inserted in the head of the inferior turbinate and advanced submucosally until the tip is beyond the middle turbinate. SITR is most commonly performed using a turbinate microdebrider device. The microdebrider blade is used to resect submucosal turbinate tissue while preserving the turbinate mucosa. Both techniques can be performed using a headlight with direct visualization or endoscopically using a rigid nasal endoscope. They can also be followed by outfracture of the turbinate which is typically performed using a Boies or Freer elevator. Complications are rare but can include epistaxis, nasal crusting and/or scarring.

While studies have demonstrated improvement in nasal obstructive symptoms after pediatric turbinate surgery, few have reported on the impact of turbinate surgery on pediatric OSA outcomes.[15–17] A retrospective study in patients with known OSA found that inferior turbinate reduction at the time of adenotonsillectomy improved physical and emotional symptoms, daytime function, and overall OSA-18 scores over adenotonsillectomy alone.[3] In a separate study in children with concurrent chronic rhinitis and OSA, turbinate reduction performed at the time of adenotonsillectomy resulted in better polysomnogram and quality-of-life outcomes than adenotonsillectomy alone.[3] Prospective, controlled trials are needed to better understand the role of pediatric turbinate surgery in both primary and persistent OSA.

Nasal Septum

The estimated prevalence of nasal septal deformity ranges from 1% to 14% in children[18,19] and is secondary to irregular development of the nasomaxillary complex or trauma.[20] Absolute indications for surgical correction of nasal septal deformity in children have traditionally included septal hematoma or abscess, nasal tumors, congenital anomalies, and severe cosmetic deformity.[21] Symptomatic nasal airway obstruction is a relative indication for septoplasty,[21] and the growing nasal airway deserves special consideration that is unique to the pediatric population.

Anthropometric studies demonstrate that the cartilaginous septum reaches near-maximal size around the age of 2 years,[22] whereas the bony septum continues to grow up to 15 years of age.[21,23] Studies of septal development in animals have raised concern that septoplasty could adversely affect mid-face and nasal growth, which has led to questions about the safety of septoplasty in young children.[24–27] In contrast, most human studies of patients who underwent septoplasty as children have demonstrated no clinically significant differences in anthropometric measurements at long-term follow-up compared to age-matched controls.[28–30]

Despite evidence that pediatric septoplasty can be performed without significant impact to nasal maturity, most authors recommend conservative techniques in this population.[27,31] The basic surgical approach is similar to that in the adult population with submucopericondrial elevation via a Killian or hemitransfixion incision.[27] Ideally, cartilage resection is targeted to the deviated part of the septum or spur, and resected segments are straightened and reimplanted when possible.[27] Incisions placed along the dorsal segment of the bony–cartilaginous junction may jeopardize dorsal height and should be avoided.[31] Furthermore, limiting mucosal elevation along the floor of the nasal cavity avoids damage to the incisive nerves.[31] In the event of nasal trauma, closed reduction can be considered to treat an acute septal fracture in a child, which is more effective in children than adults given the predominance of cartilage versus bone in the pediatric septum.[27]

There are limited data on the relationship between nasal septal deformity and OSA in children. Studies have found that subjective nasal obstruction correlates with symptoms of sleep-disordered breathing in children, and nasal septal deviation is a risk factor for persistent OSA after adenotonsillectomy.[32,33] In adults with OSA, nasal surgery can improve CPAP adherence, but has minimal effect on AHI reduction.[34,35] While data on septoplasty and pediatric OSA are lacking in children, there is evidence to support an improvement in QOL after surgical correction of symptomatic septal deformity in children.[36,37] While the revision rate for pediatric septoplasty is low at 2.9%, it is higher than in the adult population (1.1%).[38] In addition, revision cases after pediatric septoplasties are more likely to require an open septorhinoplasty.[38] These risks and benefits should be discussed with patients and families who are offered septoplasty. Risks of acquired nasal deformity and need for revision after septoplasty must be balanced with risks of leaving the crooked septum untreated in children, especially when it is a contributor to OSA.

Palate

The retropalatal airway is a common site of obstruction in OSA due to the small cross-sectional area of the velopharynx and collapsibility of the palate and lateral pharyngeal walls (**Fig. 1**).[39–41] Palatal surgery can be considered in a child with persistent OSA after adenotonsillectomy and palatal collapse on DISE.[42]

Palatal surgery aims to pull the palate forward in an anterolateral vector away from the posterior pharyngeal wall. Since the original uvulopalatopharyngoplasty (UPPP) was first described by Fujita and colleagues in 1981,[43] others have published modifications that aim to relieve obstruction while minimizing complications.[44–46] Bleeding, airway obstruction, globus pharyngeus, nasopharyngeal stenosis, and velopharyngeal insufficiency (VPI) are rare complications of palatal surgery for OSA.[44,47–49] VPI occurs in up to 8.1% of the adult population,[50] but is not well quantified in the pediatric population. More conservative, tissue-sparing surgical techniques can reduce the risk of postoperative VPI.[51] In recent decades, the expansion sphincter pharyngoplasty (ESP) has garnered favor for its more conservative, tissue-preservation approach.[11,51–53]

First described in the adult population, ESP involves transection and suture repositioning of the inferior aspect of the palatopharyngeous muscle to the hamulus, which expands the oropharyngeal airway.[54] Modifications of this technique have been described. For example, the palatopharyngeous muscles can be suspended to the periosteum of the pterygoid hamulus, the pterygomandibular raphe via a tunnel under the anterior tonsillar pillar,[55] or to the arching fibers of the palatoglossus muscle.[54] The remaining concavity between the anterior and posterior pillars is often reapproximated. Some surgeons also choose to incorporate a partial uvulectomy.

The modified ESP technique, first described by Ulualp in 2014, involves a partial thickness transection of the palatopharyngeous muscle at the upper third portion, blunt tunneling of the palate superiolaterally, and suture attachment of the isolated portion of the palatopharyngeous muscle through the tunnel to the arching fibers of the soft palate.[56] In this technique, the uvula is preserved, and the tonsillar pillars are not reapproximated. A similar procedure can be performed with barbed or non-barbed suture that travels submucosally without the need to dissect a tunnel or mobilize and transpose the posterior palatopharyngeal muscle, which can be quite thin in children. Regardless of the variation, the goal of the ESP is to open the pharyngeal airway by pulling the soft palate superiorly, anteriorly, and laterally.

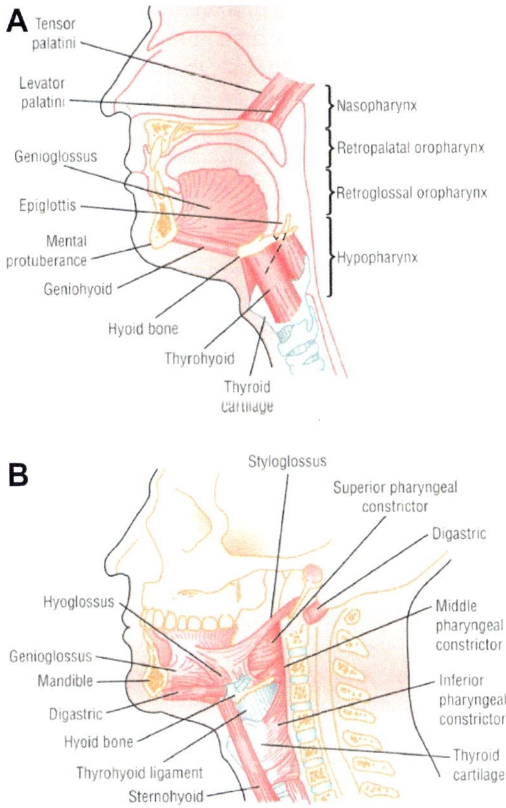

Fig. 1. Retropalatal airway. (*From* Rowley JA, Badr MS. Anatomy and Physiology of Upper Airway Obstruction. In: *Principles and Practice of Sleep Medicine*. Elsevier; 2017:1076-1087.e5. https://doi.org/10.1016/B978-0-323-24288-2.00111-2; with permission.)

There is limited literature on pediatric OSA outcomes following palatal surgery. Several early case series demonstrated improvements in AHI and O_2 nadir in children undergoing UPPP.[57–59] A retrospective review of 25 children with OSA who underwent adenotonsillectomy with palatal surgery performed via a modified ESP technique compared to 25 AHI-matched controls who underwent adenotonsillectomy alone showed a significantly lower postoperative AHI in the ESP group (mean [SD] 2.4 [3.9] versus 6.2 [6.0] events per hour; $P < .001$).[56] Furthermore, several studies have demonstrated that DISE-directed surgery, including ESP, in children with persistent OSA after adenotonsillectomy improves objective outcomes such as AHI and O_2 nadir.[60–62] A recent expert consensus statement concluded that ESP is a safe and effective management option for refractory OSA in children who demonstrate lateral pharyngeal wall collapse on DISE.[11] Further research is needed to better understand the role of palatal surgery in the management of pediatric OSA. For example, prospective randomized studies should assess whether palatal surgery at the time of adenotonsillectomy improves outcomes for children at risk for persistent OSA.

Adenoids

Adenoidectomy involves removing adenoid lymphoid tissue in the nasopharynx using a variety of techniques, such as cautery, curettage, coblation, and microdebrider resection. Although adenotonsillectomy is primary treatment for pediatric OSA, there is emerging evidence that adenoidectomy alone may be effective in treating primary OSA. For example, a recent review of children with mild OSA who underwent adenoidectomy found that only 8% of patients went on to require tonsillectomy for persistent obstruction.[63] A systematic review found that adenoidectomy alone decreased the AHI by an average of 14.4 events per hour. The authors concluded that adenoidectomy can significantly improve OSA in children and avoids the added risks of tonsillectomy.[64]

Patients with persistent OSA after adenotonsillectomy who have nasal obstruction should be evaluated for adenoid regrowth. Lateral neck radiographs and nasal endoscopy are common methods for assessing adenoid size.[65] Fortunately, symptomatic recurrent adenoid hypertrophy is uncommon and requires revision surgery in less than 2% of patients.[66,67] The mean interval between initial adenoidectomy (with or without tonsillectomy) and revision is approximately 1.5 to 3 years, with risk factors for regrowth that include eustachian tubal lymphoid hypertrophy and gastroesophageal reflux.[66,67] Further research is needed to clarify which children with primary OSA are candidates for adenoidectomy alone, as well as when revision adenoidectomy is indicated for persistent OSA.

SUMMARY

While adenotonsillectomy is the primary treatment of OSA in children, 25% to 60% of children will have persistent OSA after surgery.[11] Risk factors for persistent OSA include obesity, older age (>7 years), black race, severe preoperative OSA, trisomy 21, neuromuscular disorders, and craniofacial abnormalities.[12] Persistent OSA post-adenotonsillectomy in children should be evaluated with clinical examination and DISE to assess for additional sites of obstruction. DISE can also be used upfront in children who have severe baseline OSA or small tonsils on examination.[2] Common sources of obstruction contributing to pediatric OSA include the inferior turbinates, nasal septum, nasopharynx (eg, adenoid regrowth), and palate. There are specific surgical options available for each of the sites of obstruction.

For children with nasal obstruction and inferior turbinate hypertrophy, inferior turbinate resection can improve QOL and polysomnogram outcomes in children with OSA.[3] In children with nasal septal deformity, septoplasty can safely be performed with conservative, cartilage-sparing techniques without downstream consequences on mid-face growth. While septoplasty is associated with improved QOL outcomes, more data are needed to evaluate its association with pediatric OSA outcomes.[36,37] Anecdotally, nasal surgery in children can improve tolerance to CPAP, an effect which has been documented in adult literature. Adenoidectomy with or without tonsillectomy is the first-line treatment for pediatric OSA, but adenoid regrowth can occur and contribute to persistent symptoms.[66] This can be evaluated with nasal endoscopy in clinic or lateral neck radiographs.[65] Finally, for patients with lateral pharyngeal wall collapse on DISE, modified ESP has been shown to improve objective OSA outcomes.[56]

CLINICS CARE POINTS

- DISE has been increasingly utilized to assess for sites of obstruction in children with OSA. The nose, nasopharynx, and palate are common sites of obstruction noted on DISE in children with risk factors for post-adentonsillectomy persistence.
- Inferior turbinate reduction at the time of adenotonsillectomy may improve PSG parameters and QOL.

- Patients with persistent OSA and nasal obstruction should be evaluated for adenoid regrowth.
- Septoplasty may be appropriate for selecti children with symptomatic nasal obstruction and OSA and can be performed without downstream consequences on mid-face growth in the appropriately selected patient using conservative, cartilage-sparing techniques.
- ESP is an effective management option for children with persistent OSA after adenotonsillectomy and lateral pharyngeal wall collapse on DISE.

DISCLOSURES

E.M. Kirkham, is an author for UpToDate and is supported by the National Heart Lung and Blood Institute of the National Institutes of Health (K23HL153897). C.M. Baldassari reports involvement in the Inspire Registry. No other financial disclosures or conflicts of interest exist.

REFERENCES

1. Tauman R, Gulliver TE, Krishna J, et al. Persistence of obstructive sleep apnea syndrome in children after adenotonsillectomy. J Pediatr 2006;149(6):803–8.
2. Baldassari CM, Lam DJ, Ishman SL, et al. Expert Consensus Statement: Pediatric Drug-Induced Sleep Endoscopy. Otolaryngol Head Neck Surg 2021;165(4): 578–91.
3. Cheng PW, Fang KM, Su HW, et al. Improved objective outcomes and quality of life after adenotonsillectomy with inferior turbinate reduction in pediatric obstructive sleep apnea with inferior turbinate hypertrophy. Laryngoscope 2012;122(12):2850–4.
4. Cai Y, Goldberg AN, Chang JL. The Nose and Nasal Breathing in Sleep Apnea. Otolaryngol Clin North Am 2020;53(3):385–95.
5. Shave S, Vella J, Chandy B. Pediatric Functional Rhinoplasty. Facial Plast Surg 2023. https://doi.org/10.1055/s-0043-1772576.
6. Sullivan S, Li K, Guilleminault C. Nasal obstruction in children with sleep-disordered breathing. Ann Acad Med Singap 2008;37(8):645–8.
7. Cao Y, Wu S, Zhang L, et al. Association of allergic rhinitis with obstructive sleep apnea: A meta-analysis. Medicine (Baltim) 2018;97(51):e13783.
8. Johnson C, Leavitt T, Daram SP, et al. Obstructive Sleep Apnea in Underweight Children. Otolaryngol Head Neck Surg 2022;167(3):566–72.
9. Li HY, Lin Y, Chen NH, et al. Improvement in quality of life after nasal surgery alone for patients with obstructive sleep apnea and nasal obstruction. Arch Otolaryngol Head Neck Surg 2008;134(4):429–33.
10. Ishii L, Roxbury C, Godoy A, et al. Does Nasal Surgery Improve OSA in Patients with Nasal Obstruction and OSA? A Meta-analysis. Otolaryngol Head Neck Surg 2015;153(3):326–33.
11. Ishman SL, Maturo S, Schwartz S, et al. Expert Consensus Statement: Management of Pediatric Persistent Obstructive Sleep Apnea After Adenotonsillectomy. Otolaryngol Head Neck Surg 2023;168(2):115–30.
12. Kirkham EM. Pediatric Drug-Induced Sleep Endoscopy. Otolaryngol Clin North Am 2022;55(6):1165–80.
13. Wilcox LJ, Bergeron M, Reghunathan S, et al. An updated review of pediatric drug-induced sleep endoscopy. Laryngoscope Investig Otolaryngol 2017;2(6): 423–31.

14. Ng DK, hong Chan C, yan Hwang GY, et al. A review of the roles of allergic rhinitis in childhood obstructive sleep apnea syndrome. Allergy Asthma Proc 2006;27(3): 240–2.
15. Komshian SR, Cohen MB, Brook C, et al. Inferior Turbinate Hypertrophy: A Review of the Evolution of Management in Children. Am J Rhinol Allergy 2019; 33(2):212–9.
16. Whelan RL, Shaffer AD, Stapleton AL. Efficacy of inferior turbinate reduction in pediatric patients: a prospective analysis. Int Forum Allergy Rhinol 2021; 11(12):1654–62.
17. Manzi B, Sykes KJ, Wei JL. Sinonasal Quality of Life in Children After Outfracture of Inferior Turbinates and Submucous Inferior Turbinoplasty for Chronic Nasal Congestion. JAMA Otolaryngol Head Neck Surg 2017;143(5):452–7.
18. Podoshin L, Gertner R, Fradis M, et al. Incidence and treatment of deviation of nasal septum in newborns. Ear Nose Throat J 1991;70(8):485–7.
19. Song SY, Kim IT, Chang KH, et al. The Prevalence of Nasal Septal Deformities among Children in Kindergarten and First Grade in Anyang and Kunpo Cities. J Rhinol 1999;6(1):58–60.
20. Zielnik-Jurkiewicz B, Olszewska-Sosińska O. The nasal septum deformities in children and adolescents from Warsaw, Poland. Int J Pediatr Otorhinolaryngol 2006;70(4):731–6.
21. Justicz N, Choi S. When Should Pediatric Septoplasty Be Performed for Nasal Airway Obstruction? Laryngoscope 2019;129(7):1489–90.
22. Van Loosen J, Van Zanten GA, Howard CV, et al. Growth characteristics of the human nasal septum. Rhinology 1996;34(2):78–82.
23. Akgüner M, Barutçu A, Karaca C. Adolescent growth patterns of the bony and cartilaginous framework of the nose: a cephalometric study. Ann Plast Surg 1998;41(1):66–9.
24. Sarnat BG, Wexler MR. Growth of the face and jaws after resection of the septal cartilage in the rabbit. Am J Anat 1966;118(3):755–67.
25. Meeuwis J, Verwoerd-Verhoef HL, Verwoerd CD. Normal and abnormal nasal growth after partial submucous resection of the cartilaginous septum. Acta Otolaryngol 1993;113(3):379–82.
26. Siegel MI. A Longitudinal Study of Facial Growth in Papio cynocephalusafter Resection of the Cartilagenous Nasal Septum. J Med Primatol 1979;8(2):122–7.
27. Christophel JJ, Gross CW. Pediatric Septoplasty. Otolaryngol Clin 2009;42(2): 287–94.
28. Tasca I, Compadretti GC. Nasal growth after pediatric septoplasty at long-term follow-up. Am J Rhinol Allergy 2011;25(1):e7–12.
29. El-Hakim H, Crysdale WS, Abdollel M, et al. A Study of Anthropometric Measures Before and After External Septoplasty in Children: A Preliminary Study. Arch Otolaryngol Head Neck Surg 2001;127(11):1362.
30. Walker PJ, Crysdale WS, Farkas LG. External Septorhinoplasty in Children: Outcome and Effect on Growth of Septal Excision and Reimplantation. Arch Otolaryngol Head Neck Surg 1993;119(9):984–9.
31. Cingi C, Muluk NB, Ulusoy S, et al. Septoplasty in children. Am J Rhinol Allergy 2016;30(2):e42–7.
32. Fernandes M de BL, Salgueiro AGNS, Bighetti EJB, et al. Symptoms of Obstructive Sleep Apnea, Nasal Obstruction, and Enuresis in Children With Nonsyndromic Cleft Lip and Palate: A Prevalence Study. Cleft Palate Craniofac J 2019; 56(3):307–13.

33. Guilleminault C, shu HY, Glamann C, et al. Adenotonsillectomy and obstructive sleep apnea in children: a prospective survey. Otolaryngol Head Neck Surg 2007;136(2):169–75.
34. Friedman M, Tanyeri H, Lim JW, et al. Effect of improved nasal breathing on obstructive sleep apnea. Otolaryngol Head Neck Surg 2000;122(1):71–4.
35. Wu J, Zhao G, Li Y, et al. Apnea-hypopnea index decreased significantly after nasal surgery for obstructive sleep apnea: A meta-analysis. Medicine (Baltim) 2017;96(5):e6008.
36. Yilmaz MS, Guven M, Akidil O, et al. Does septoplasty improve the quality of life in children? Int J Pediatr Otorhinolaryngol 2014;78(8):1274–6.
37. Lee VS, Gold RM, Parikh SR. Short-term quality of life outcomes following pediatric septoplasty. Acta Otolaryngol 2017;137(3):293–6.
38. Shah JP, Youn GM, Wei EX, et al. Septoplasty Revision Rates in Pediatric vs Adult Populations. JAMA Otolaryngol Head Neck Surg 2022;148(11):1044–50.
39. Ayappa I, Rapoport DM. The upper airway in sleep: physiology of the pharynx. Sleep Med Rev 2003;7(1):9–33.
40. Schwab RJ, Gupta KB, Gefter WB, et al. Upper airway and soft tissue anatomy in normal subjects and patients with sleep-disordered breathing. Significance of the lateral pharyngeal walls. Am J Respir Crit Care Med 1995;152(5 Pt 1):1673–89.
41. Trudo FJ, Gefter WB, Welch KC, et al. State-related changes in upper airway caliber and surrounding soft-tissue structures in normal subjects. Am J Respir Crit Care Med 1998;158(4):1259–70.
42. Sharma AV, Padhya T, Nallu S. Management of Pediatric Obstructive Sleep Apnea After Failed Tonsillectomy and Adenoidectomy. Adv Pediatr 2022;69(1): 95–105.
43. Fujita S, Conway W, Zorick F, et al. Surgical correction of anatomic azbnormalities in obstructive sleep apnea syndrome: uvulopalatopharyngoplasty. Otolaryngol Head Neck Surg 1981;89(6):923–34.
44. MacKay SG, Carney AS, Woods C, et al. Modified uvulopalatopharyngoplasty and coblation channeling of the tongue for obstructive sleep apnea: a multicentre Australian trial. J Clin Sleep Med 2013;9(2):117–24.
45. Neruntarat C. Uvulopalatal flap for obstructive sleep apnea: short-term and long-term results. Laryngoscope 2011;121(3):683–7.
46. Tanyeri H, Polat S, Kirişoğlu CE, et al. Long-term efficacy of submucosal uvulopalatopharyngoplasty for obstructive sleep apnea syndrome. Eur Arch Oto-Rhino-Laryngol 2012;269(9):2069–74.
47. Kezirian EJ, Weaver EM, Yueh B, et al. Incidence of serious complications after uvulopalatopharyngoplasty. Laryngoscope 2004;114(3):450–3.
48. Kandasamy T, Wright ED, Fuller J, et al. The incidence of early post-operative complications following uvulopalatopharyngoplasty: identification of predictive risk factors. J Otolaryngol Head Neck Surg 2013;42(1):15.
49. Camacho M, Certal V, Modi R, et al. Tissue-Sparing Uvulopalatopharyngoplasty for OSA: Conservative, Compassionate and Possibly just as Effective. Indian J Otolaryngol Head Neck Surg 2019;71(1):5–6.
50. Tang JA, Salapatas AM, Bonzelaar LB, et al. Long-Term Incidence of Velopharyngeal Insufficiency and Other Sequelae following Uvulopalatopharyngoplasty. Otolaryngol Head Neck Surg 2017;156(4):606–10.
51. Ehsan Z, Ishman SL. Pediatric Obstructive Sleep Apnea. Otolaryngol Clin North Am 2016;49(6):1449–64.
52. Smith DF, Sa T, Fenchel M, et al. Temporal trends in inpatient pediatric sleep apnea surgery: 1993-2010. Laryngoscope 2017;127(5):1235–41.

53. Cohn JE, Relyea GE, Daggumati S, et al. Multilevel Sleep Surgery Including the Palate in Nonsyndromic, Neurologically Intact Children with Obstructive Sleep Apnea. OTO Open 2019;3(2). 2473974X19851473.
54. Pang KP, Woodson BT. Expansion Sphincter Pharyngoplasty: A New Technique for the Treatment of Obstructive Sleep Apnea. Otolaryngol Head Neck Surg 2007;137(1):110–4.
55. Hong SN, Kim HG, Han SY, et al. Indications for and Outcomes of Expansion Sphincter Pharyngoplasty to Treat Lateral Pharyngeal Collapse in Patients With Obstructive Sleep Apnea. JAMA Otolaryngol Head Neck Surg 2019;145(5):405–12.
56. Ulualp SO. Modified expansion sphincter pharyngoplasty for treatment of children with obstructive sleep apnea. JAMA Otolaryngol Head Neck Surg 2014; 140(9):817–22.
57. Kerschner JE, Lynch JB, Kleiner H, et al. Uvulopalatopharyngoplasty with tonsillectomy and adenoidectomy as a treatment for obstructive sleep apnea in neurologically impaired children. Int J Pediatr Otorhinolaryngol 2002;62(3):229–35.
58. Marcus CL, Brooks LJ, Draper KA, et al. Diagnosis and Management of Childhood Obstructive Sleep Apnea Syndrome. Pediatrics 2012;130(3):576–84.
59. Com G, Carroll JL, Tang X, et al. Characteristics and surgical and clinical outcomes of severely obese children with obstructive sleep apnea. J Clin Sleep Med 2015;11(4):467–74.
60. He S, Peddireddy NS, Smith DF, et al. Outcomes of Drug-Induced Sleep Endoscopy-Directed Surgery for Pediatric Obstructive Sleep Apnea. Otolaryngol Head Neck Surg 2018;158(3):559–65.
61. Wootten CT, Chinnadurai S, Goudy SL. Beyond adenotonsillectomy: outcomes of sleep endoscopy-directed treatments in pediatric obstructive sleep apnea. Int J Pediatr Otorhinolaryngol 2014;78(7):1158–62.
62. Esteller E, Villatoro JC, Agüero A, et al. Outcome of drug-induced sleep endoscopy-directed surgery for persistent obstructive sleep apnea after adenotonsillar surgery. Int J Pediatr Otorhinolaryngol 2019;120:118–22.
63. Volsky PG, Woughter MA, Beydoun HA, et al. Adenotonsillectomy vs Observation for Management of Mild Obstructive Sleep Apnea in Children. Otolaryngol Head Neck Surg 2014;150(1):126–32.
64. Reckley LK, Song SA, Chang ET, et al. Adenoidectomy can improve obstructive sleep apnoea in young children: systematic review and meta-analysis. J Laryngol Otol 2016;130(11):990–4.
65. Baldassari CM, Choi S. Assessing adenoid hypertrophy in children: X-ray or nasal endoscopy? Laryngoscope 2014;124(7):1509–10.
66. Grindle CR, Murray RC, Chennupati SK, et al. Incidence of revision adenoidectomy in children. Laryngoscope 2011;121(10):2128–30.
67. Monroy A, Behar P, Brodsky L. Revision adenoidectomy–a retrospective study. Int J Pediatr Otorhinolaryngol 2008;72(5):565–70.

Surgical Management of Pediatric Obstructive Sleep Apnea Beyond Tonsillectomy & Adenoidectomy: Tongue Base and Larynx

Matthew Maksimoski, MD[a], Carol Li, MD[b,*]

KEYWORDS

- Lingual tonsillectomy • Tongue base suspension • Geniohyoid advancement
- Supraglottoplasty • Epiglottopexy • Posterior midline glossectomy

KEY POINTS

- Sleep endoscopy and/or cross-sectional dynamic imaging should be used to evaluate sites of upper airway obstruction in the surgical evaluation of children with persistent obstructive sleep apnea (OSA).
- The tongue base is one of the most common areas of obstruction in children with persistent OSA after adenotonsillectomy.
- Surgery of the tongue base includes lingual tonsillectomy, posterior midline glossectomy, and less commonly tongue or hyoid suspension.
- Supraglottoplasty and epiglottopexy can address laryngeal obstruction leading to persistent OSA.
- Postoperative complications that can arise following tongue base and laryngeal surgery include bleeding, edema, oropharyngeal stenosis, and dysphagia.

EPIDEMIOLOGY

The success rates of adenotonsillectomy for pediatric obstructive sleep apnea (OSA) range from 66% to 79% for patients without significant comorbidities, while those with medical comorbidities have success rates on the order of 40%.[1,2] After adenotonsillectomy, the tongue base is the most common primary source of obstruction in children; it has been identified in 35% to 85%.[3–5] Special consideration is given to

[a] Division of Pediatric Otolaryngology, Cincinnati Children's Hospital Medical Center, 3333 Burnet Avenue, MLC 2018, Cincinnati, OH 45229, USA; [b] Division of Pediatric Otolaryngology, Department of Otolaryngology–Head and Neck Surgery, University of Cincinnati College of Medicine, Cincinnati Children's Hospital Medical Center, 3333 Burnet Avenue, MLC 2018, Cincinnati, OH 45229, USA
* Corresponding author.
E-mail address: carol.li@cchmc.org

Otolaryngol Clin N Am 57 (2024) 431–445
https://doi.org/10.1016/j.otc.2024.02.005
0030-6665/24/

children with Trisomy 21, who have lingual tonsil hypertrophy (35%) much more commonly than nonsyndromic populations (3%).[6] Lingual tonsillectomy is the most common surgery performed for children with persistent OSA following adenotonsillectomy.[7,8] Reports of other surgical procedures, such as posterior midline glossectomy (PMG), epiglottopexy, hyoid suspension, and geniohyoid advancement, are scant in the pediatric population and clinical outcomes are not well studied.

RELEVANT ANATOMY AND PHYSIOLOGY

The tongue base and larynx are involved in swallowing, breathing, and speaking. The oropharynx includes the tongue base and lingual tonsil tissue up to the vallecula while the laryngeal surface of the epiglottis and arytenoid tissue are part of the larynx. The aryepiglottic folds are considered "marginal" in their position between the oropharynx and the larynx, and are generally considered a part of the larynx and hypopharynx.

The lingual tonsil is the inferior most portion of the lymphoid tissue within the oropharynx, and forms the inferior border of "Waldeyer's ring". The lingual tonsil tissue extends from the base of tongue's posterior surface into the vallecula[9] and is graded from 1 to 4 according to the bulk and degree of obstruction[9,10] (**Fig. 1**).

The tongue base is composed of musculature with overlying mucosa and lingual tonsils. Within the tongue itself are the lingual nerve branches and the lingual artery.[9] Extrinsic tongue muscles, most pertinently the geniohyoid, digastric (anterior belly), and mylohyoid muscles, create tension on the hyoid bone anteriorly to the inferior border of the mandible. Inferiorly, the thyrohyoid and sternohyoid musculature allows for depression of the hyoid bone. The stylohyoid muscle pulls the hyoid and tongue base posterosuperiorly. These muscles act in concert to physiologically move the tongue base through manipulation of the floating hyoid bone.[9,11] Upper airway obstruction and OSA due to tongue base obstruction can be due to an enlarged tongue (macroglossia), retropositioning of the base of tongue (glossoptosis), or both.

PREOPERATIVE EVALUATION

Patients with persistent sleep symptoms after adenotonsillectomy should undergo polysomnography to determine the presence of persistent OSA and diagnostic studies to evaluate secondary sites of obstruction and identify those which may be amenable to surgical treatment.[12,13] Persistent OSA should be addressed in a shared decision-making model using an interdisciplinary approach as management can include both medical and surgical options. Evaluation by specialists from sleep

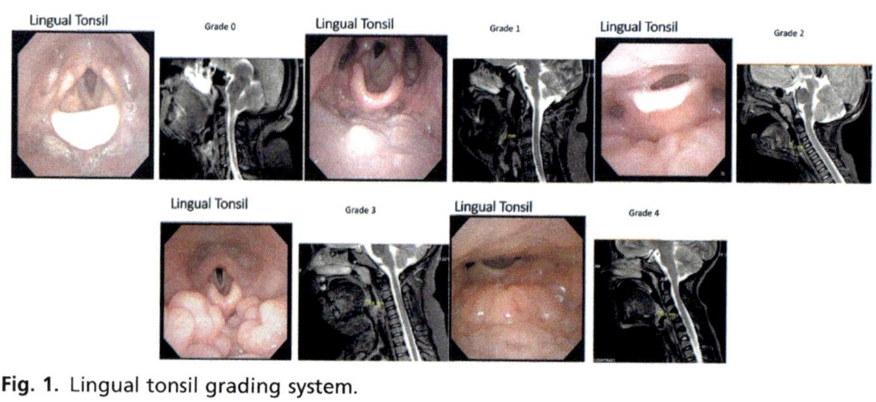

Fig. 1. Lingual tonsil grading system.

medicine, otolaryngology, pulmonology, oromaxillofacial surgery, plastic surgery, nutrition, and behavioral psychology may be necessary.

To identify additional surgical targets, a careful physical examination and additional diagnostic procedures, such as sleep endoscopy and/or dynamic cross-sectional imaging, should be performed to evaluate sites of upper airway obstruction. Multiple areas of obstruction are often identified, including locations in the larynx and/or tongue base. While multisite surgery may be tempting to avoid the need for multiple anesthetics especially in the pediatric population, there is a some risk of oropharyngeal scarring and stenosis.[14] Therefore, this senior author recommends staged surgeries when multiple sites of obstruction need to be addressed.

Surgery of the tongue base and the larynx should be performed if it is identified as the primary level of obstruction. When tongue base or larynx is determined to be secondary, it does not seem to affect surgical failure rates when surgery is undertaken only on the primary site of obstruction. Previous studies showed no difference in surgical success when a secondary lesion of the nasopharynx, oropharynx, or larynx was present but not addressed.[15,16] Additional anatomic considerations such as retrognathia, micrognathia, trismus, oropharyngeal stenosis, and vascular malformations of the tongue base should be identified prior to surgery as they may impact the safety and success of the procedure[17] (**Fig. 2**).

Surgery of the larynx and the tongue base can affect voice and swallowing function.[18] For patients with baseline dysphagia and/or those at high risk for swallowing dysfunction, swallow evaluation should be performed prior to surgical intervention.[18] Caution should be taken not to be overly aggressive in tissues resection in order to minimize the risk of aspiration and dysphagia.[19]

SURGICAL TECHNIQUES

Lingual Tonsillectomy

Indications and preoperative considerations

Lingual tonsil hypertrophy is the most common cause of obstruction in patients with persistent OSA after adenotonsillectomy.[7,8] Care should be taken during endoscopic evaluation of the tongue base as lingual tonsil size can be overestimated in patients with a thin layer of lingual tonsil overlying a prominent tongue base. Cross-sectional imaging such as MRI or intraoperative evaluation of the tongue base can be employed for further differentiation between lingual tonsil tissue and tongue base musculature.[5,16] Palpation and manipulation of the base of tongue to feel for softer lymphoid tissue rather than firmer muscle may also be helpful if imaging studies are not readily available (**Fig. 3**).

Operative technique

Owing to the risk of bleeding and edema, the procedure is performed under general anesthesia with endotracheal intubation. Although a nasotracheal tube is preferred by some to optimize full visualization of the surgical field, an orotracheal tube is preferred by others to elevate the palate. Long-acting paralytic agents should not be utilized as stimulation of tongue musculature with cautery can be used to gauge depth of dissection during lingual tonsil removal.[20]

An operating laryngoscope (eg, Lindholm or Parsons) in or out of suspension can be employed for adequate exposure of lingual tonsil tissue. Of note, consideration should be given to risk of spinal cord compression in patients with Trisomy 21 due to atlantoaxial instability. In this population, suspension can be avoided or lessened to keep the neck in a neutral position. Suspension can also be performed with the use of a tonsil retractor such as a Crowe–Davis or McIvor retractor. A silk suture is often passed

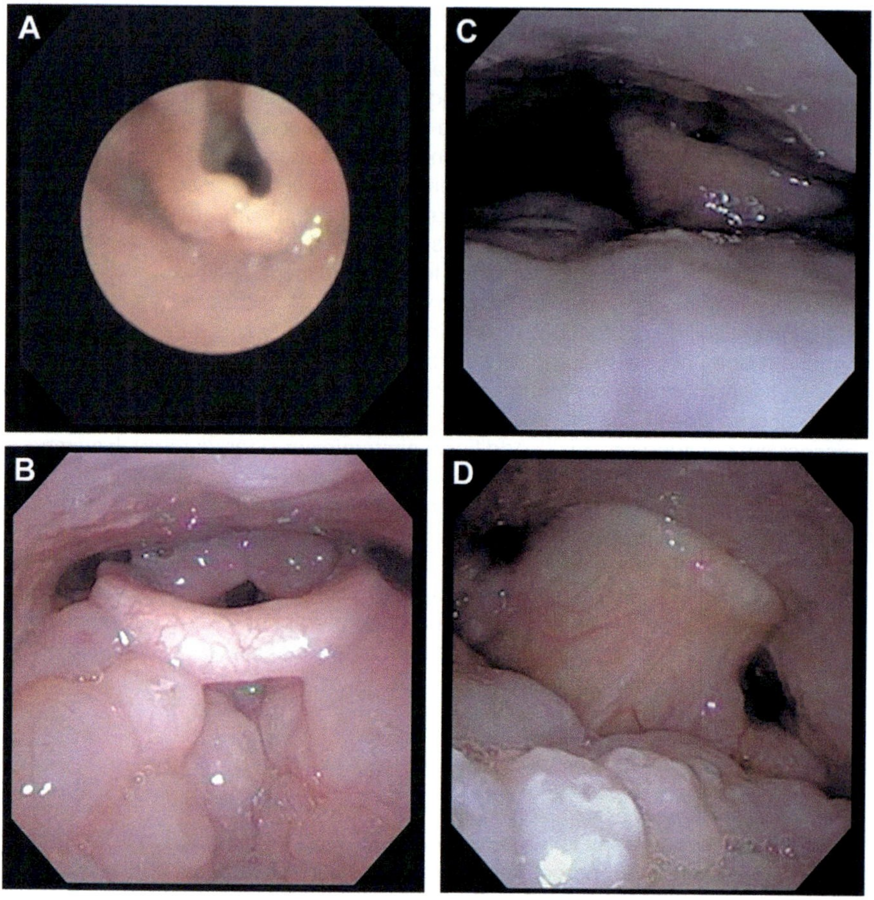

Fig. 2. Areas of obstruction at the level of the tongue base and the larynx which may be visualized on DISE. (*A*) Laryngomalacia, (*B*) lingual tonsil hypertrophy, (*C*) tongue base collapse without lingual tonsil hypertrophy, (*D*) epiglottic prolapse without base of tongue collapse.

through the midline of the tongue anteriorly for traction especially when a laryngoscope is not employed. A telescope (straight or angled) or an operating microscope can be used to visualize the tongue base. The benefits of suspension include an ability to work bimanually and obtain a close view of the tongue base, along with the ability to photo-document the procedure. Drawbacks of suspension include the inability to manipulate the tongue or change exposure without releasing the suspension. If the patient is not placed in suspension, a large laryngoscope can be inserted into the oropharynx and swept back and forth throughout the case for visualization or a telescope can be used with tongue retraction. Benefits to this technique include the ability to readily change exposure of the lymphoid tissue throughout the case. Drawbacks include the need for a single-handed technique and inability to use a microscope.

Radiofrequency ablation can be used to excise tissue while optimizing hemostasis. A suction monopolar cautery can also be used to ablate and suction the lymphoid tissue although is slower. The microdebrider technique has also been described and may allow for faster removal of tissue, though electrocautery is necessary for hemostasis.

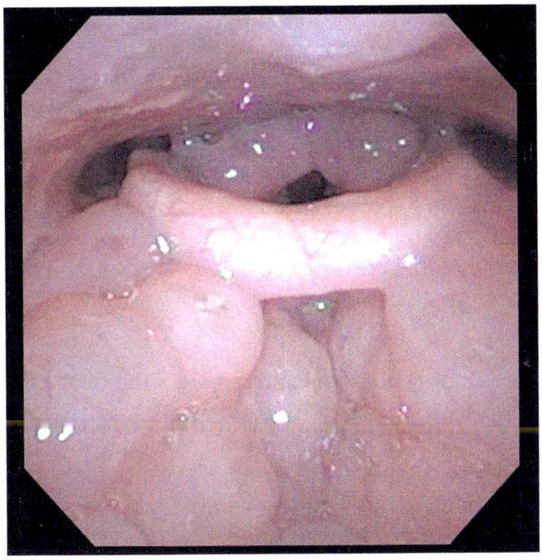

Fig. 3. Lingual tonsil hypertrophy as visualized on DISE.

If the patient is placed in suspension, timing should be noted to ensure the suspension is relaxed and the tongue allowed to reperfuse at least once per hour.[8,20–22] Regardless of the instrument used, the aim of the surgery should be to remove lingual tonsil tissue down to the level of the basement membrane overlying the base of tongue musculature. Special attention should be paid to removing lingual tonsil tissue which may exist inferiorly in the vallecula and lead to retroflexion of the epiglottis.

After full removal of the lingual tonsil tissue, close examination should be taken to view the lateral recesses of the glossotonsillar sulcus bilaterally to ensure there is no remnant tissue. The patient may then be extubated per the institution's protocols (**Fig. 4**).

Complications

Bleeding, as with palatine tonsil bleeding, can be a significant issue after lingual tonsillectomy. One single institutional series identified a bleeding rate of 4.4% (defined as any blood visualized by the family) and noted this was similar to the risk of bleeding from adenotonsillectomy.[21]

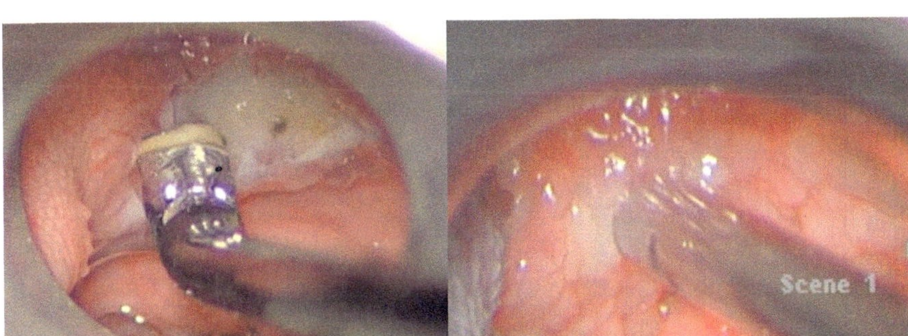

Fig. 4. Lingual tonsillectomy as performed with radiofrequency ablation (*left*) and microdebrider (*right*).

Injury to the epiglottis can occur during removal of the inferior extent of the lingual tonsil tissue, which can lead to scarring, aspiration, and pain. If there is concern for bleeding from the epiglottis, consideration should be given to using topical vasoconstrictors for hemostasis rather than cauterization techniques.

In a 2010 single institutional series of 49 patients, they noted that when lingual tonsillectomy is performed with additional oropharyngeal surgery, oropharyngeal scarring occurred in 4 of 49 (8.2%)[14]; however, subsequent studies have not found this to be the case if care is taken to minimize continguous raw surfaces in this area. The addition of laryngeal surgery (eg, supraglottoplasty or epiglottopexy) has not been shown to results in oropharyngeal scarring.[23]

Surgical outcomes

Overall, lingual tonsillectomy outcomes are some of the best defined of sleep surgery. Meta-analyses support a success rate (postoperative apnea-hypopnea index [AHI] < 5) of 52% and a mean reduction in AHI of 6.6 events per hour[7,8]; with preoperative oAHI ranging from 8.5 to 18.3 events per hour and postoperative oAHI ranging from 3.2 to 9.7 events per hour. Overall, studies with a baseline higher preoperative oAHI reported larger reductions in oAHI with one study reporting a reduction in oAHI from a mean of 81.4 to 40.9 and a second from 8.51 to 4.07.[24,25]

Posterior Midline Glossectomy

Indications and preoperative considerations

Patients with anterior–posterior collapse of the tongue base on drug-induced sleep endoscopy (DISE) may be candidates for a PMG. Discussion should be undertaken with the patient and their family to review other possible options such as tongue suspension or hypoglossal nerve stimulation depending on candidacy factors (**Fig. 5**).

Operative technique

Similar to lingual tonsillectomy, patients may be orally or nasotracheally intubated. While it is not performed universally in primary surgery, it is the practice of the authors'

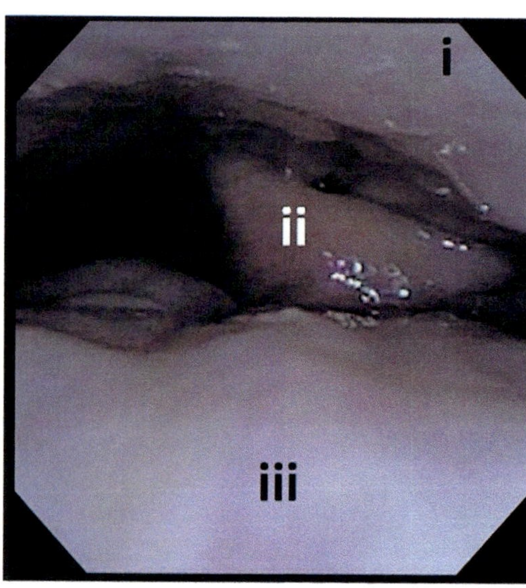

Fig. 5. Independent posterior tongue base collapse without lingual tonsil hypertrophy: (i) Posterior pharyngeal wall, (ii) epiglottis, and (iii) tongue base.

institution to perform ultrasound of the tongue base prior to the start of the procedure to determine the course of the lingual arteries. Lateral distance from the midline and depth from the mucosa are commonly measured at 2 points in the posterior tongue (1–2 cm anterior to the circumvallate papillae and a second point posteriorly) to approximate a safe area for dissection.[26] Computed tomographic angiography has also been described for this purpose.[27] When ultrasound is not used, cadaveric studies show that a 1 cm width for excision can typically be used safely, even with traction on the tongue.[28] Long-term paralytic agents should be avoided to allow for indication of proximity to the lingual arteries and overlying lingual nerves. Local anesthesia with lidocaine or bupivacaine with epinephrine can be injected submucosally into the midline posteriorly in the surgical field.

The surgery may be performed endoscopically with the use of an angled scope and radiofrequency ablation or electrocautery to remove the midline portion of the tongue. Alternatively, PMG can be performed through direct visualization with exposure of the tongue base using a mouth gag (eg, Jennings gag) and a midline tongue suture for anterior retraction. The senior author's technique is to create a midline mucosal incision with needle-point cautery starting 1 to 2 cm anterior to the circumvallate papillae and extend posteriorly. The incision is then deepened using radiofrequency ablation, while creating lateral mucosal flaps. Retraction sutures (3-0 silk) are placed in the elevated mucosal flaps for visualization.[20,29,30] The needle-point cautery and radiofrequency wand are used in an alternating manner to extend the mucosal incision posteriorly and ablate tongue musculature, respectively. The total length of the excised area should extend from just anterior to the circumvallate papillae to above the lingual–epiglottic ligament.[20,30] When adequate tissue has been removed, the anterior aspect of the mucosal incision is closed with absorbable sutures, with an open area posteriorly to allow for drainage (**Fig. 6**).

Complications

There are few reports of complications after PMG in children but 2 studies have reported that bleeding is a less frequent occurrence with PMG compared to lingual tonsillectomy, which may be due to the closure performed after PMG leaving a smaller raw surface.[29,31] However, bleeding from PMG may be higher volume than lingual tonsillectomy as they more commonly involve the dorsal lingual artery. Dysphagia has been reported, and pain leading to poor oral intake, both at rates less than 10%[30,31] (**Fig. 7**).

Surgical outcomes

Outcomes from PMG are not as well published as those from lingual tonsillectomy or supraglottoplasty, but in those studies with reported polysomnographic outcomes, rates of surgical success range from 46% to 87%, with AHI improvements from 2.6 to 41.3 events per hour. Preoperative oAHI ranged from 5.23 to 48.6 and postoperative oAHI ranged from 2.68 to 34.1.[20,27,29–31] However, caution should be exercised when interpreting these data due to the small sample size of the currently available literature. Surgical success is defined in a variable manner in these studies, some defined it as postoperative oAHI less than 5, while others followed clinical symptoms, and one study did not define the measure of success.

Epiglottopexy

Indications and preoperative considerations

Patients with independent prolapse of the epiglottis during DISE may be candidates for epiglottopexy. Because epiglottic prolapse can be secondary to collapse of the tongue base and/or lingual tonsil hypertrophy, differentiating obstruction that is

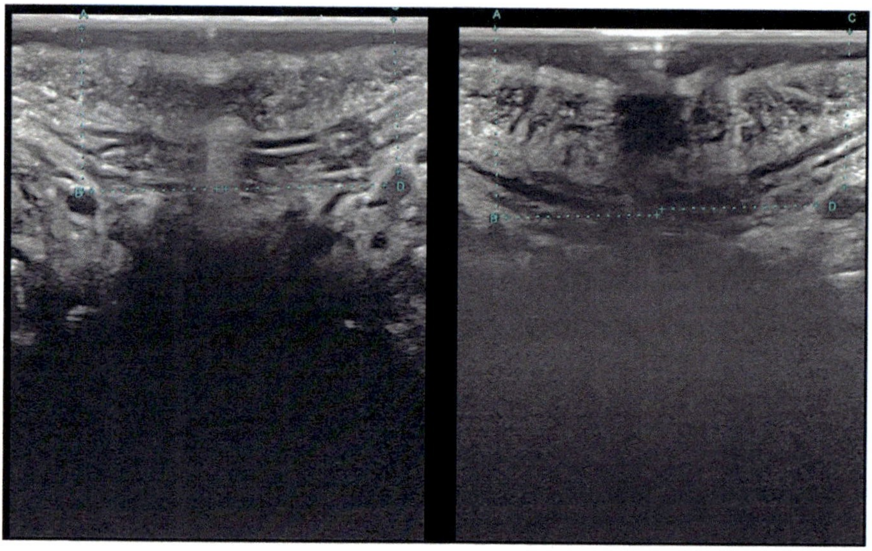

Fig. 6. Sonographic imaging of the lingual arteries prior to posterior midline glossectomy with both anterior (*left*) and posterior (*right*) windows. Right lingual artery: Depth from the tongue surface: 9.4 m (anterior), 11.0 mm (posterior); distance from the midline: 7.4 mm (anterior), 9.0 mm (posterior). Left lingual artery: Depth from the tongue surface: 8.7 m (anterior), 9.1 mm (posterior); distance from the midline: 9.2 mm (anterior), 9.2 mm (posterior).

primarily due to tongue base prolapse is important to determine which surgery is most likely to address the collapse[23,32] (**Fig. 8**).

Operative technique

Epiglottopexy is typicically performed transorally either under spontaneous ventilation or with intubation. This senior author prefers spontaneous ventilation to avoid endotracheal intubation if tolerated by the patient to allow for ease of instrumentation within the endolaryngeal space during suture placement. The patient is placed in suspension with an operating laryngoscope to expose the lingual surface of the epiglottis, the vallecula, and the posteroinferior portion of the base of tongue in the midline. The glossoepiglottic ligament should be readily identified. With the use of cold instrumentation,

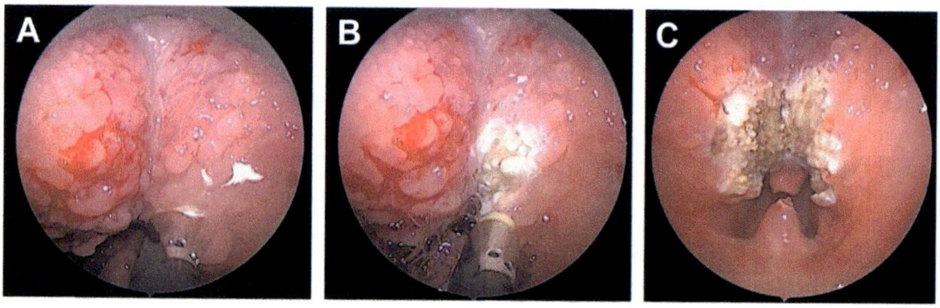

Fig. 7. Posterior midline glossectomy, performed via endoscopic approach through the mouth: (*A*) Initial incision, (*B*) development of the trough; and (*C*) final resection cavity.

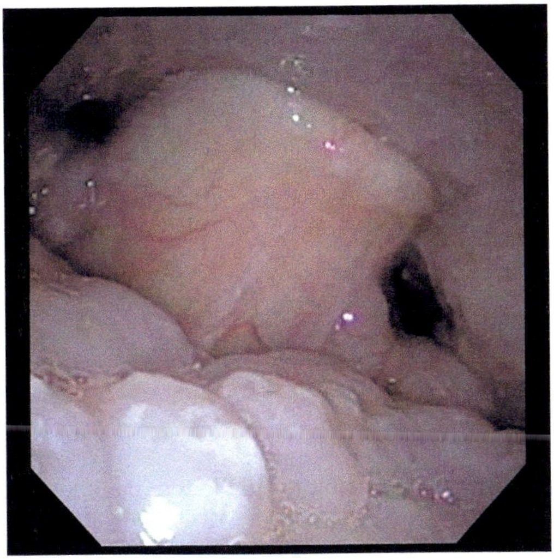

Fig. 8. Independent epiglottic prolapse on DISE.

CO_2 laser, or radiofrequency ablation, the base of tongue along the vallecula and the lingual surface of the epiglottis are denuded of mucosa to create opposing raw surfaces while leaving the mucosa intact on the superior surface of the epiglottis. At this point, the lingual–epiglottic ligament is shortened and tightened with either monopolar or bipolar cautery. A suture is usually passed through the soft tissue of the tongue base and through the lingual surface of the epiglottis, taking care to not violate the laryngeal surface. The suture should ideally pass partially through the epiglottic cartilage to provide an adequate purchase to hold the epiglottis in place. Quantities of suture of 1, 3, and 5 sutures have been described as standard practice based on the institution. Publications describe the use of both vicryl (Ethicon) and PDS (Ethicon) sutures, usually 4-0 or 5-0 in diameter.[23,32–35] The suture is then tied down and the patient emerged from anesthesia. Less frequently, some surgeons rely on the scarring between the denuded surface to form the bond between the epiglottis and tongue base (**Fig. 9**).

Complications

As with any manipulation of the larynx, postoperative edema can lead to airway obstruction so all reports of the procedure advocate for overnight observation. Owing to the small area of surgical intervention, bleeding has not been a reported complication. Dysphagia is a concern with manipulation of the epiglottis as with the tongue base procedures above and one study did note transient odynophagia in 2 patients.[23] Reports published of epiglottopexy advocate for a clinical evaluation of swallowing at minimum with many describing standard instrumental swallow evaluation with either flexible endoscopic evaluation of swallowing (FEES) or video fluoroscopic swallow study (VFSS).[23,32,34]

Many concerns exist for the suturing of the epiglottis to the tongue base as in the case of epiglottopexy, and the concern for new onset dysphagia is a frequent topic of discussion at national meetings when the procedure is discussed. Although multiple studies have been published on the safety of epiglottopexy and lack of new-onset dysphagia,[23,32–36] no randomized trials exist and a high degree of clinical suspicion is paramount to prevent new swallowing problems after surgery.

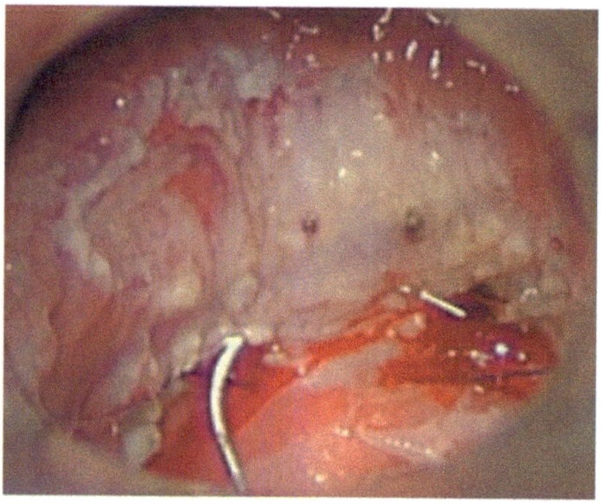

Fig. 9. Endoscopic suturing of the epiglottis to the tongue base in epiglottopexy

Surgical outcomes

Success rates for epiglottopexy are not as well established as other procedures due to small case series, but all series report a less than 70% success rate, congruent with other DISE-directed surgeries.[23,32–36] Total reduction in oAHI ranges from 3.9 to 9.0 events per hour in those studies reporting outcomes.[23,36] Unfortunately, the definition of surgical success is not standardized in epiglottopexy publications, with some using AHI less than 5 or greater than 50% reduction in AHI,[23] others using clinical resolution of stridor,[33] some using AHI less than 10,[36] and others following clinical appearance.[32,35]

Supraglottoplasty

Indications and preoperative considerations

Unlike congenital or feeding-variant laryngomalacia, sleep-variant laryngomalacia can present later in life and may not be readily visualized without performing sleep endoscopy. Additional sites of airway obstruction should be evaluated as laryngomalacia is reported to be associated with a secondary level of obstruction in up to 64% of cases[37,38] (**Fig. 10**).

Operative technique

When tolerated, the senior author prefers to perform supraglottoplasty with the patient under spontaneous ventilation although intubation does allow for extension of the aryepiglottic folds and may allow for more additional operative time. Following application of topical anesthesia, the larynx is exposed with an operating laryngoscope or telescope. The aryepiglottic fold is divided up to the level of the false vocal folds. This can be performed bilaterally either with cold instrumentation or a laser. If redundant arytenoid mucosa exists which appears to be contributing to the laryngeal obstruction, it can be removed by grasping the superior redundant mucosa and excising it or using a microdebrider. Care should be taken to leave a bridge of tissue between the trimmed aryepiglottic fold and the excised tissue to prevent scarring. Several other methods using the microdebrider, radiofrequency ablation, and even sinus true cuts have also been described[39,40] (**Fig. 11**).

Complications

Complications from supraglottoplasty are relatively rare and it is well tolerated by most patients. Bleeding has rarely been reported, but as with all laryngeal surgeries, dysphagia is a risk. Studies generally report rates of new postoperative dysphagia

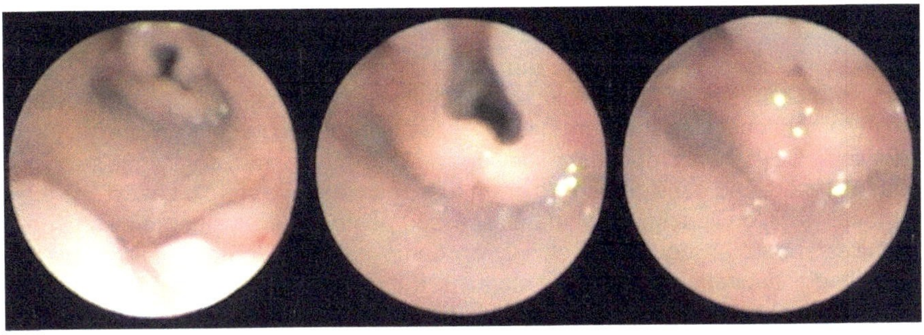

Fig. 10. Laryngomalacia as viewed on DISE.

less than 5%,[11] and of those with immediate postoperative dysphagia, 75% showed resolution 14 months after surgery.[42]

Surgical outcomes

Multiple studies have shown the success of supraglottoplasty for treatment of OSA, with one meta-analysis showing an average reduction from a preoperative AHI of 14.0 to 3.3 events per hour.[43] Another systematic review showed an average reduction in oAHI of 21.0 with DISE-directed supraglottoplasty, utilizing a different set of studies than the previous one.[44,45] Overall rates of success (final oAHI < 5) range from 60% to 72% depending on the study.[43,46] Supraglottoplasty is supported as standard of care for patients with evidence of laryngomalacia and apneas.[18]

Additional Surgical Techniques

Several other surgical techniques may be used by the experienced practitioner in the pediatric patient with refractory OSA after adenotonsillectomy. Owing to a paucity of evidence in the pediatric population or rare usage, these are not discussed in detail in this article. Some of these procedures include hyoid suspension, which has been discussed in the adult population[47] and anecdotally used in pediatric patients. Another technique is tongue-base suspension, in which the suture is passed through the soft tissue of the tongue rather than around the hyoid bone. Evidence in the pediatric population is limited with only one case series[48] and one case report.[49] Finally, vocal fold immobility can also airway obstruction resulting in OSA and a wide range of surgical techniques can be considered in the appropriate patient.

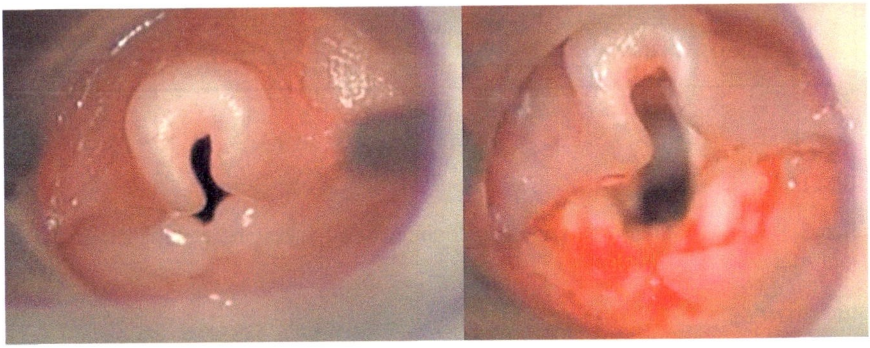

Fig. 11. Laryngomalacia of the larynx before (*left*) and after (*right*) undergoing supraglottoplasty.

POSTOPERATIVE CARE

Surgery of the tongue base and the larynx is generally performed with an overnight observation. While same-day discharge after supraglottoplasty has been described, many practitioners feel there are insufficient data to support its safety, especially in children with OSA. Owing to the risk of airway swelling, intraoperative systemic steroids are often utilized, and consideration is given to a postoperative steroid course.[5,8,17,30]

Ideall, swallow function should be assessed postoperatively prior to discharge and families should be counseled closely on complications such as swelling, bleeding, dysphagia, aspiration, and airway stenosis. If there are any concerns for new aspiration or dysphagia, FEES or VFSS should be considered.[32,36]

Following tongue base or endolaryngeal sleep surgery, patients should undergo a postoperative sleep study and symptom screen to evaluate for persistent OSA which may have been incompletely addressed.

SUMMARY

The tongue base and the larynx are common sites of upper airway obstruction in children with persistent OSA following adenotonsillectomy. In the pediatric population, surgical management of the tongue base and the larynx can include lingual tonsillectomy, PMG, supraglottoplasty, and epiglottopexy. Short-term complications of surgery include airway edema and bleeding. Patients are typically observed in the hospital overnight following surgery. More rare complications to consider after tongue base and laryngeal procedures include dysphagia and aspiration. Therefore, swallow function should be evaluated pre- and postoperatively especially in high-risk patients. Although large volume studies are limited, current evidence shows that surgery of the tongue base and the larynx can provide significant benefit to the management of OSA in appropriately selected patients.

CLINICS CARE POINTS

- Children with persistent sleep disturbance following adenotonsillectomy should undergo evaluation with polysomnography.
- Additional sites of upper airway obstruction can be identified using drug-induced sleep endoscopy and/or dynamic cross-sectional imaging such as cine MRI.
- The lingual tonsils and tongue base are common sites of obstruction in children with persistent OSA following adenotonsillectomy.
- Various upper airway procedures that target the tongue base and larynx exist to treat persistent OSA in children.

DISCLOSURE

Drs C. Li and M. Maksimoski have no financial or other disclosures relative to the subject matter of this article.

REFERENCES

1. Marcus CL, Moore RH, Rosen CL, et al. A randomized trial of adenotonsillectomy for childhood sleep apnea. N Engl J Med 2013;368(25):2366–76.

2. Friedman M, Wilson M, Lin HC, et al. Updated systematic review of tonsillectomy and adenoidectomy for treatment of pediatric obstructive sleep apnea/hypopnea syndrome. Otolaryngol Head Neck Surg 2009;140(6):800–8.
3. Ehsan Z, Ishman SL. Pediatric Obstructive Sleep Apnea. Otolaryngol Clin North Am 2016;49(6):1449–64.
4. Wilcox LJ, Bergeron M, Reghunathan S, et al. An updated review of pediatric drug-induced sleep endoscopy. Laryngoscope Investig Otolaryngol 2017;2(6): 423–31.
5. Isaiah A, Kiss E, Olomu P, et al. Characterization of upper airway obstruction using cine MRI in children with residual obstructive sleep apnea after adenotonsillectomy. Sleep Med 2018;50:79–86.
6. Fricke BL, Donnelly LF, Shott SR, et al. Comparison of lingual tonsil size as depicted on MR imaging between children with obstructive sleep apnea despite previous tonsillectomy and adenoidectomy and normal controls. Pediatr Radiol 2006;36(6):518–23.
7. Manickam PV, Shott SR, Boss EF, et al. Systematic review of site of obstruction identification and non-CPAP treatment options for children with persistent pediatric obstructive sleep apnea. Laryngoscope 2016;126(2):491–500.
8. Rivero A, Durr M. Lingual Tonsillectomy for Pediatric Persistent Obstructive Sleep Apnea: A Systematic Review and Meta-analysis. Otolaryngol Head Neck Surg 2017;157(6):940–7.
9. Lesperance MM, Flint PW. Cummings pediatric otolaryngology. Philadelphia: Elsevier Saunders; 2015. p. 411, xii.
10. Friedman M, Yalamanchali S, Gorelick G, et al. A standardized lingual tonsil grading system: interexaminer agreement. Otolaryngol Head Neck Surg 2015; 152(4):667–72.
11. Flint PW, Haughey BH, Lund VJ, et al. Cummings otolaryngology-head and neck surgery. 7. Philadelphia: Elsevier; 2020. volumes cm p.
12. Baldassari CM, Lam DJ, Ishman SL, et al. Expert consensus statement: Pediatric drug-induced sleep endoscopy. Otolaryngol Head Neck Surg 2021;165(4): 578–91.
13. Ishman SL, Maturo S, Schwartz S, et al. Expert consensus stement: Management of pediatric persistent obstructive sleep apnea after adenotonsillectomy. Otolaryngol Head Neck Surg 2023;168(2):115–30.
14. Prager JD, Hopkins BS, Propst EJ, et al. Oropharyngeal stenosis: a complication of multilevel, single-stage upper airway surgery in children. Arch Otolaryngol Head Neck Surg 2010;136(11):1111–5.
15. Michelson AP, Hawley K, Anne S. Do synchronous airway lesions predict treatment failure after adenotonsillectomy in children less than 3 years of age with obstructive sleep apnea? Int J Pediatr Otorhinolaryngol 2014;78(9):1439–43.
16. Boudewyns A, Verhulst S, Maris M, et al. Drug-induced sedation endoscopy in pediatric obstructive sleep apnea syndrome. Sleep Med 2014;15(12):1526–31.
17. Wootten CT, Shott SR. Evolving therapies to treat retroglossal and base-of-tongue obstruction in pediatric obstructive sleep apnea. Arch Otolaryngol Head Neck Surg 2010;136(10):983–7.
18. Carter J, Rahbar R, Brigger M, et al. International Pediatric ORL Group (IPOG) laryngomalacia consensus recommendations. Int J Pediatr Otorhinolaryngol 2016;86:256–61.
19. Lawlor CM, Choi S. Diagnosis and Management of Pediatric Dysphagia: A Review. JAMA Otolaryngol Head Neck Surg 2020;146(2):183–91.

20. Woodson BL S. Lingual tonsillectomy and midline posterior glossectomy for obstructive sleep apnea. Operat Tech Otolaryngol Head Neck Surg 2012;23(2): 155–61.
21. DeMarcantonio MA, Senser E, Meinzen-Derr J, et al. The safety and efficacy of pediatric lingual tonsillectomy. Int J Pediatr Otorhinolaryngol 2016;91:6–10.
22. Kang KT, Koltai PJ, Lee CH, et al. Lingual Tonsillectomy for Treatment of Pediatric Obstructive Sleep Apnea: A Meta-analysis. JAMA Otolaryngol Head Neck Surg 2017;143(6):561–8.
23. Maksimoski M, Maurrasse SE, Hoff SR, et al. Pediatric sleep outcomes after endoscopy-directed simultaneous lingual tonsillectomy and epiglottopexy. J Otolaryngol Head Neck Surg 2022;51(1):11.
24. Lin AC, Koltai PJ. Persistent pediatric obstructive sleep apnea and lingual tonsillectomy. Otolaryngol Head Neck Surg 2009;141(1):81–5.
25. Wootten CT, Chinnadurai S, Goudy SL. Beyond adenotonsillectomy: outcomes of sleep endoscopy-directed treatments in pediatric obstructive sleep apnea. Int J Pediatr Otorhinolaryngol 2014;78(7):1158–62.
26. Liu C, Qin J, Xing D, et al. Ultrasonic Measurement of Lingual Artery and Its Application for Midline Glossectomy. Ann Otol Rhinol Laryngol 2020;129(9):856–62.
27. Li S, Shi H. Lingual artery CTA-guided midline partial glossectomy for treatment of obstructive sleep apnea hypopnea syndrome. Acta Otolaryngol 2013;133(7): 749–54.
28. Ye J, Wang J, He L, et al. [Anatomic characteristics of lingual artery and midline glossectomy]. Zhonghua Er Bi Yan Hou Ke Za Zhi 2001;36(1):55–7.
29. Propst EJ, Amin R, Talwar N, et al. Midline posterior glossectomy and lingual tonsillectomy in obese and nonobese children with down syndrome: Biomarkers for success. Laryngoscope 2017;127(3):757–63.
30. Dorrity J, Wirtz N, Froymovich O, et al. Genioglossal Advancement, Hyoid Suspension, Tongue Base Radiofrequency, and Endoscopic Partial Midline Glossectomy for Obstructive Sleep Apnea. Otolaryngol Clin North Am 2016;49(6): 1399–414.
31. Williamson A, McArdle EH, Morrow VR, et al. Base of Tongue Surgery and Pediatric Obstructive Sleep Apnea. Otolaryngol Head Neck Surg 2023;168(4):839–47.
32. Oomen KP, Modi VK. Epiglottopexy with and without lingual tonsillectomy. Laryngoscope 2014;124(4):1019–22.
33. Whymark AD, Clement WA, Kubba H, et al. Laser epiglottopexy for laryngomalacia: 10 years' experience in the west of Scotland. Arch Otolaryngol Head Neck Surg 2006;132(9):978–82.
34. Werner JA, Lippert BM, Dunne AA, et al. Epiglottopexy for the treatment of severe laryngomalacia. Eur Arch Oto-Rhino-Laryngol 2002;259(9):459–64.
35. Schraff SADD. Labioglossopexy and epiglottopexy. Operat Tech Otolaryngol Head Neck Surg 2005;259:459–64.
36. Kanotra SP, Givens VB, Keith B. Swallowing outcomes after pediatric epiglottopexy. Eur Arch Oto-Rhino-Laryngol 2020;277(1):285–91.
37. Dickson JM, Richter GT, Meinzen-Derr J, et al. Secondary airway lesions in infants with laryngomalacia. Ann Otol Rhinol Laryngol 2009;118(1):37–43.
38. Landry AM, Thompson DM. Laryngomalacia: disease presentation, spectrum, and management. Int J Pediatr 2012;2012:753526.
39. Groblewski JC, Shah RK, Zalzal GH. Microdebrider-assisted supraglottoplasty for laryngomalacia. Ann Otol Rhinol Laryngol 2009;118(8):592–7.

40. El-Sobki A, Ibrahim RAE, Amer A, et al. Coblation supraglottoplasty: a ten-year experience in a tertiary referral hospital. Eur Arch Oto-Rhino-Laryngol 2022; 279(2):865–74.
41. Eustaquio M, Lee EN, Digoy GP. Feeding outcomes in infants after supraglottoplasty. Otolaryngol Head Neck Surg 2011;145(5):818–22.
42. Nguyen M, Brooks L, Wetzel M, et al. Swallowing Outcomes Following Supraglottoplasty: A Retrospective Review. Laryngoscope 2021;131(12):2817–22.
43. Camacho M, Dunn B, Torre C, et al. Supraglottoplasty for laryngomalacia with obstructive sleep apnea: A systematic review and meta-analysis. Laryngoscope 2016;126(5):1246–55.
44. Lee CF, Hsu WC, Lee CH, et al. Treatment outcomes of supraglottoplasty for pediatric obstructive sleep apnea: A meta-analysis. Int J Pediatr Otorhinolaryngol 2016;87:18–27.
45. Farhood Z, Ong AA, Nguyen SA, et al. Objective Outcomes of Supraglottoplasty for Children With Laryngomalacia and Obstructive Sleep Apnea: A Meta-analysis. JAMA Otolaryngol Head Neck Surg 2016;142(7):665–71.
46. Chan DK, Truong MT, Koltai PJ. Supraglottoplasty for occult laryngomalacia to improve obstructive sleep apnea syndrome. Arch Otolaryngol Head Neck Surg 2012;138(1):50–4.
47. Bowden MT, Kezirian EJ, Utley D, et al. Outcomes of hyoid suspension for the treatment of obstructive sleep apnea. Arch Otolaryngol Head Neck Surg 2005; 131(5):440–5.
48. Hartzell LD, Guillory RM, Munson PD, et al. Tongue base suspension in children with cerebral palsy and obstructive sleep apnea. Int J Pediatr Otorhinolaryngol 2013;77(4):534–7.
49. Valika T, Maksimoski M, Maurrasse S. Pediatric Tongue Base Suspension With Fluoroscopic Guidance. Laryngoscope 2021;131(9):2112–4.

Neurostimulation for Pediatric Obstructive Sleep Apnea

Doug Chieffe, MD[a], Christopher Hartnick, MD, MS[a,b,c,*]

KEYWORDS

- Pediatric obstructive sleep apnea • Down syndrome • Upper airway stimulation

KEY POINTS

- Hypoglossal nerve stimulation/upper airway stimulation (UAS) is an emerging therapy for children with Down syndrome and persistent obstructive sleep apnea after adenotonsillectomy.
- Several modifications to current adult UAS pathways must be made to account for challenges inherent to caring for a complex pediatric population, including patient selection, surgical technique, perioperative care, and postimplantation device programming.
- Drug-induced sleep endoscopy is essential to patient selection in UAS and must be performed and recorded in a systematic manner.
- Modifications must be made to surgical techniques used in adults in order to account for challenges unique to children with DS, including patient positioning, incision planning, and post-operative care.
- Device programming is essential for ensuring optimal outcomes. Modification must be made to existing programming protocols used in adults.

INTRODUCTION

Up to 80% of children with Down syndrome (DS) are affected by obstructive sleep apnea (OSA), which has deleterious effects on cardiopulmonary function, neurocognition, and quality of life.[1–3] The American Academy of Otolaryngology recommends adenotonsillectomy (T&A) as the first-line treatment of children with OSA.[4] However, only 16% to 33% of children with DS will have resolution of OSA with T&A.[5–8] This low response rate may be attributed to complex multilevel airway obstruction in DS; children with DS often have additional sites of obstruction, such as the tongue

[a] Otolaryngology–Head and Neck Surgery, Massachusetts Eye and Ear Infirmary, 243 Charles Street, Boston, MA 02114, USA; [b] Division of Pediatric Otolaryngology, Pediatric Airway, Voice, and Swallowing Center; [c] Harvard Medical school, Boston, MA, USA
* Corresponding author. Otolaryngology–Head and Neck Surgery, Massachusetts Eye and Ear Infirmary, 243 Charles Street, Boston, MA 02114.
E-mail address: christopher_hartnick@meei.harvard.edu

Otolaryngol Clin N Am 57 (2024) 447–455
https://doi.org/10.1016/j.otc.2024.02.007

base.[9] Additional surgical intervention may be necessary in children with DS and persistent OSA, as only 50% of such children will tolerate positive airway pressure therapy.[10]

Hypoglossal nerve stimulation, or upper airway stimulation (UAS), is a well-established treatment of adults with OSA and was recently approved by the Food and Drug Administration (FDA) for treatment of children with DS and persistent OSA following T&A who meet specific inclusion and exclusion criteria.[11–13] The original trial for UAS in adults demonstrated a 75% response rate with a favorable risk profile.[11] We have previously reported the safety and efficacy of UAS in children with DS and persistent OSA after T&A in a study that included 12 months of follow-up.[12] Our study found a similar therapeutic response and adverse event profile to adults, with a 65.9% response rate. Additionally, 77.9% of pediatric patients with DS had moderate-to-large improvements in validated quality of life measures.

There are well-established protocols for activation and titration of the device following surgical implantation in adult patients with OSA. However, given the challenges associated with caring for a complex pediatric population, these protocols cannot be directly applied to children with DS. This article will review patient selection, operative technique, postoperative care, and postimplantation optimization in children with DS.

THE FOOD AND DRUG ADMINISTRATION CANDIDACY

Children aged 13 to 18 years with DS and persistent severe OSA after T&A can be considered for UAS. To be eligible, their apnea-hypopnea index (AHI) must be 10 to 50 with less than 25% of the total apnea index comprised of central or mixed apnea events. In addition, patients must be continuous positive airway pressure intolerant. In patients that meet the aforementioned criteria, a drug-induced sleep endoscopy (DISE) should be performed to confirm the presence of tongue base collapse that improves with jaw thrust and to assess for unfavorable patterns of collapse such as complete concentric collapse (CCC) at the level of the soft palate, which is a current contraindication to UAS.

It is important to note that although body mass index (BMI) criteria is not specified in the recent FDA approval for pediatric DS UAS, there are no data on efficacy in children with BMI greater than 95th percentile (based on Centers for Disease Control and Prevention neurotypical growth curves) as obese children were excluded from the initial trial. Obese adults are not typically considered candidates for UAS, which is in part due to the increased likelihood of them having CCC on DISE. Assessing UAS in the obese DS pediatric population will be an important area to focus on for future research as many patients with DS fall into the obese category.

DRUG-INDUCED SLEEP ENDOSCOPY

DISE is a diagnostic procedure that evaluates the sites of obstruction while under sedation and is a critical component of patient selection for UAS. The goal of performing a DISE is to (1) ensure that there are no other surgically correctable sites of collapse such as residual adenoid tissue, prominent lingual tonsils, or certain patterns of velar or oropharyngeal collapse and (2) determine candidacy for UAS (confirm tongue base collapse without CCC).

As discussed earlier, CCC is considered a contraindication to UAS. Early studies in adults demonstrated that patients who had CCC on DISE had a worse response to UAS.[14,15] Emerging data in adult UAS literature have also suggested that patients with lateral oropharyngeal collapse may have poorer outcomes than those with anterior posterior palatal collapse or tongue base collapse.[16] Although the pathophysiology for these observations is still being investigated, studies have shown that UAS predominantly increases airway diameter in the anterior–posterior dimension.[17] Thus, many sleep surgeons recommend performing a palatoplasty prior to UAS in patients with lateral oropharyngeal collapse or CCC.

Numerous protocols, grading systems, and pharmacologic regimens have been published for pediatric DISE; however, no single protocol is uniformly accepted. A recent consensus statement on pediatric DISE called for a pediatric protocol that could be widely adopted to standardize evaluation and treatment algorithms.[18] This topic is covered elsewhere in this issue; however, several points are worth emphasizing here as DISE is central to insurance coverage of UAS.

It is essential to systematically evaluate and record each of the following sites for at least 2 to 5 breathing cycles: anterior nasal cavity, adenoids/nasopharynx (from the Mueller position), velum, oropharynx (observe lateral walls and, if present, tonsils), tongue base, epiglottis/supraglottis, and trachea (if symptoms suggest lower airway pathology such as stridor or cough). The degree of collapse (which can be reported as a percentage or absent/partial/complete) and pattern of collapse (anterior–posterior, lateral, or concentric) are noted for each level. The scope is then retracted to the level of the tongue base and velum, and the effects of a jaw thrust are observed.

SURGICAL TECHNIQUE

A complete review of the surgical technique is beyond the scope of this article. However, several key points will be discussed here.

Positioning

DS is associated with atlantoaxial instability, and as such, the neck should be kept in a neutral, nonextended position throughout the procedure. This positioning restriction significantly constrains exposure, necessitates placing the incision higher than in an adult, and places the marginal mandibular nerve at higher risk of traction injury.

Incision Planning

The traditional surgical approach involved 3 incisions—a right submental incision for stimulation lead placement, a second just below the clavicle for implantable pulse generator (IPG) placement, and a third in the midaxillary line between the fifth and sixth ribs for the sensing lead.[19] In 2018, we modified our surgical approach to eliminate the superior chest incision traditionally used to place the IPG.[20] This served to move the incision away from the IPG pocket, reducing stress on the incision (given the smaller chest wall to distribute tension), and reduced the number of incisions to be picked at.

Recently, a different 2-incision approach has been adopted in the adult population.[21,22] In this approach, the IPG and sensing lead are placed through an incision centered over the second to fifth rib. Compared to our 2-incision approach, this requires significantly less tunneling through the soft tissue of the chest wall and obviates prolonged arm immobilization with a shoulder sling. However, we take caution in universally adopting this approach in children not only for the previously cited concern regarding tension from the bulk of the IPG, but also the potential for creating breast deformities in developing female individuals. Incisions through developing breast buds can result in hypoplasia and creates fibrosis between breast tissue and the chest wall, both of which can lead to significant contour deformities.[23] Other authors have proposed additional modifications to improve cosmesis by avoiding incisions over the breast.[24] We counsel families on the risks and benefits of each approach and make a shared decision on the optimal approach for each child and family.

Postoperative Dressing

The majority of wound complications in our cohort was attributed to chronic picking. Wound care can be challenging in this population, as there is a high rate of sensory processing disorders. In order to prevent picking at the surgical site, we place a multilayer dressing in the operating room consisting of Steri-strips, Telfa, Tegaderm, and a compressive dressing. The compressive dressing is removed on post-operative day 1 (POD 1), and the remaining dressing is allowed to fall off on its own.

Additionally, if the IPG is placed through a low chest wall incision (our original 2-incision approach), which involves extensive tunneling, it is important to restrict the use of the arm to prevent the migration of the IPG and sense lead. Similar to wound care, it can be difficult to maintain activity restrictions on arm use in children. As such, we instruct the family to keep a shoulder sling in place for 4 weeks postoperatively. We have not seen device migration yet.

Postoperative Pain Management

Pain is notoriously difficult to assess in individuals with DS. Traditionally, it was thought that individuals with DS have a higher threshold for pain. However, numerous studies have disproved this notion and describe the difficulties in assessing pain in this population.[25] It is difficult to assess pain in children with DS because they not only have differing abilities to verbalize pain, but they are also often slower to display behavioral and physiologic signs of pain.[25] Parents and family members may be the best to assess pain levels but may still underestimate the degree of pain being experienced.[25] Early in our experience, we relied on acetaminophen and ibuprofen to treat pain. However, many families have self-connected through a Facebook group (Adolescents with Down Syndrome and Hypoglossal Nerve Stimulator) and their experiences have informed many modifications to the perioperative care of these children. With this feedback, we currently use acetaminophen and ketorolac scheduled every 8 hours for 5 days postoperatively with anecdotally better pain control.

POSTIMPLANTATION OPTIMIZATION

Although the success of the device is related, in part, to patient-related factors, device programming is essential to ensuring optimal outcomes.[14–16,26] The primary device parameter that is modified is the stimulation threshold. Understimulation results in subtherapeutic treatment, and overstimulation may cause sleep disturbances and result in worsened sleep. There are well-established protocols for device activation in adult patients with OSA. In the current adult protocols, the functional threshold (FT) of the device is estimated in clinic with the patient awake approximately 4 weeks after implantation. The device is then programmed using the FT, and the patient self-titrates their device until the first postimplantation polysomnogram (PSG), which is typically performed 3 months postoperatively. This allows the patient to habituate to the sensation of the device prior to evaluating and titrating the effect on sleep. However, the approach to activation and titration is more challenging in children with DS as they often have difficulty reporting the effects of different stimulation levels, which increases the risk of understimulation or overstimulation during this period. Additionally, the high rate of sensory processing disorders complicates the process of habituating the patient to stimulation, and underscores the importance of avoiding discomfort from overstimulation.

Currently, there is variation in activation practices among the few centers that provide UAS to children with DS. At our center, the first device activation occurs during a PSG so the device can be titrated to optimal effect without causing sleep disruption. Other centers mirror the adult protocol and program the device based on clinical estimations of FT and allow the family to titrate the device at home for 4 to 6 weeks prior to the first PSG. Repeat PSGs are obtained every 6 months until optimal performance is obtained.

Activation Visit

A clinic visit is scheduled for the afternoon before the first PSG. During the visit, the surgical sites are examined to ensure adequate healing. A physician programmer is then used to obtain an FT (the lowest voltage that results in protrusion of the tongue) and ensure the sense lead waveform is adequate.

The FT is estimated by having the patient gently open their mouth and serially increase stimulation from the sensation level by 0.1 V until the tongue protrudes, typically just up to or past the lower teeth. In children that are unable to hold their mouth open long enough for assessment of FT, the neck will be examined for "bull frogging" as a signal of the functional level (**Fig. 1**).

The sense lead waveform should also be examined at the activation visit to ensure the lead did not migrate during healing. An ideal sense lead waveform has good rise and fall, with inspiration being on the top half of the waveform (**Fig. 2**).

Acclimation Polysomnogram

The ultimate goal of UAS is to titrate to an AHI less than 5 in pediatric patients with DS; however, titration should be a gradual process to allow the patient time to habituate to the sensation of stimulation. The aim of the initial PSG (termed the acclimation PSG) is to identify a level of stimulation that does not cause arousals or discomfort and that leads to some improvement in obstruction. Attempting to eliminate all snoring and respiratory events at this point will likely lead to overstimulation as the patient has not yet acclimated to the sensation of stimulation. To achieve this, the initial stimulation level should be set to 0.2 V below the FT determined during the daytime activation visit

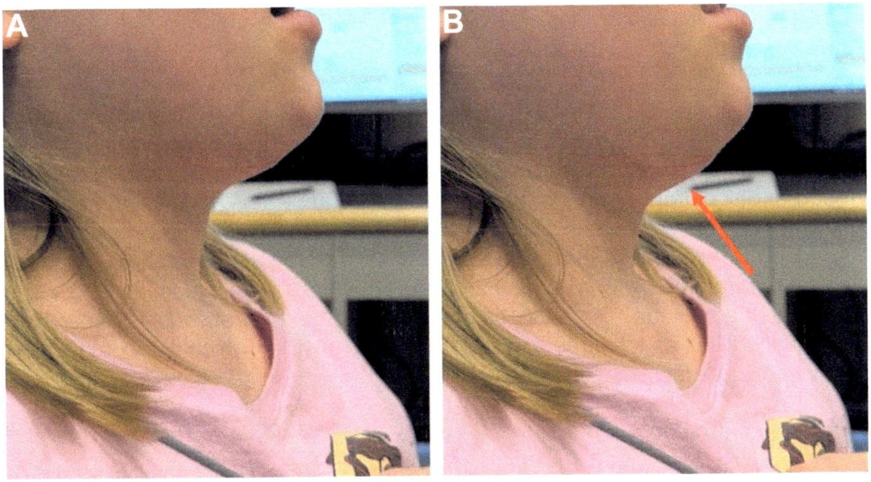

Fig. 1. Demonstration of "bull frogging." There is an increased submental fullness (*red arrow*) with the device on (*B*) compared with the device off (*A*).

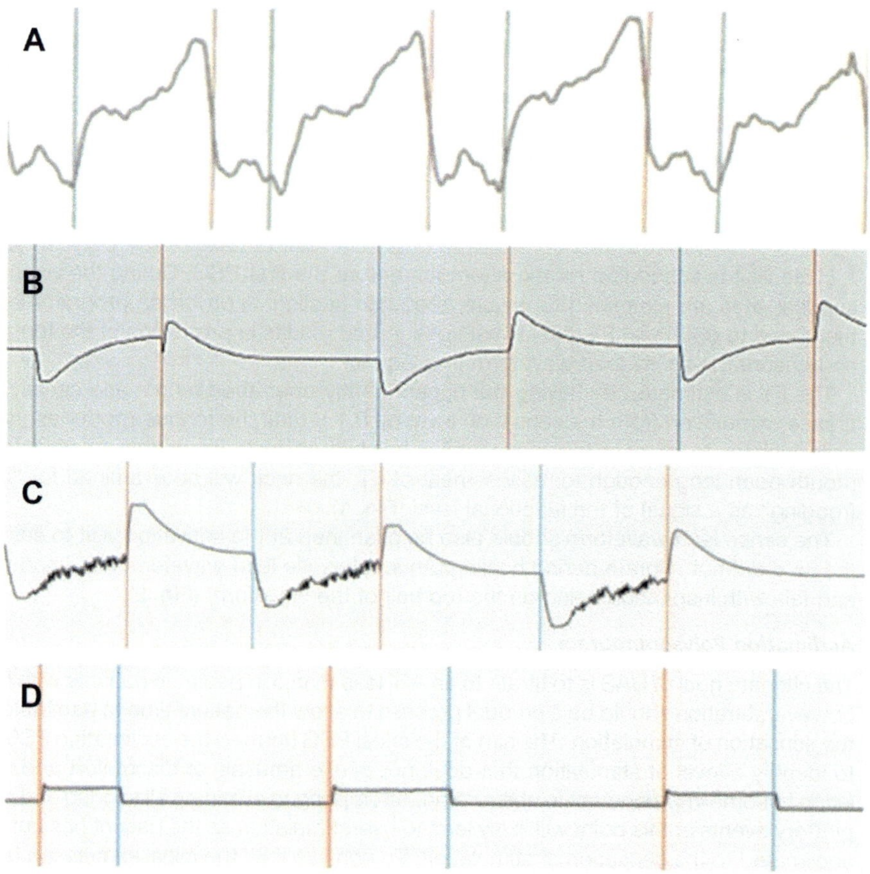

Fig. 2. (*A*) A normal sensing waveform. Note good rise and fall of the waveform coinciding with patient respiration. (*B*) Mechanical waveform indicating incomplete sense lead insertion into IPG. (*C*) High-frequency artifact indicates failure at the distal sense lead. (*D*) Flat waveform showing no rise and fall as well as sharp, downward deflections when stimulation turns on.

(same day as this PSG). If the FT is unknown, start at 1.0 V. The stimulation should be increased by 0.1 to 0.2 V no faster than every 10 to 20 minutes if AHI is greater than 10. The stimulation is decreased by 0.2 V if any of the following are observed: patient report of discomfort, or arousals related to device activation. At the end of the acclimation PSG, the device should be programmed to the lowest titrated amplitude that reduced the AHI to less than 10/h and was comfortable for the patient. The device is then programmed with a range 0.2 V below the titrated amplitude, and 0.5 V above the titrated amplitude. The patient's caregiver can then increase their stimulation by 0.1 V each week as tolerated until they see their provider (which is recommended to be 4 weeks postacclimation PSG).

Titration Polysomnograms

PSGs after the acclimation PSG are termed titration PSGs. During the initial safety and efficacy trial, titration PSGs were performed at 2, 6, and 12 months postoperatively. There is not currently a consensus on the timing of titration PSGs, but they should be obtained at least every 6 months until optimal performance is achieved. Titration PSGs follow the same protocol as the acclimation protocol; however, some centers increase stimulation by no more than 0.3 to 0.5 V per PSG while others do not have titration limits.

While long-term findings and outcomes in pediatric UAS patients are still limited, the repeat PSGs should be obtained every 2 years for the first 5 years postoperatively to ensure ongoing efficacy as the child grows and potentially undergoes changes in body habitus.

Advanced Settings

In some UAS patients, an optimal setting cannot be determined by titrating the stimulation amplitude alone (typically, the only setting evaluated during initial titration PSGs). In such cases, additional device parameters can be modified to improve performance. These settings can be modified during awake endoscopy, DISE, or a PSG, and include electrode configuration, pulse width and rate, timing settings (start delay, pause time, and therapy duration), and sensing settings to improve stimulation synchronization with respiration. These advanced settings are valuable when treating this complex population but require an in-depth knowledge of the device programming and should only be done in coordination with individuals experienced in this area including device manufacturer representatives and experienced, certified UAS surgeons.

If advanced programming is needed, a DISE can be scheduled within 1 month of a PSG with poor efficacy. During the DISE, the effect of various advanced programming changes can be evaluated, as well as the effect of different body and neck positions, and the effect of jaw thrust with and without stimulation. A PSG 1 to 2 months later would be utilized to assess improvement in efficacy and evaluate additional advanced settings. Of note, sensing settings should only be evaluated during an advanced PSG with an Inspire representative present to achieve optimal results.

SUMMARY

UAS is a promising therapy for children with DS and persistent OSA after T&A. There is robust experience with UAS in adults; however, protocols for adults cannot be directly applied to children with DS and must be modified to take into account the challenges inherent to this complex pediatric population. Future research is needed in many areas to optimize candidacy criteria (ie, role of BMI and other collapse patterns) and post-implantation programming.

CLINICS CARE POINTS

- Hypoglossal nerve stimulation, or UAS, was recently approved by the FDA for treatment of children with DS and persistent OSA following T&A.
- DISE is essential to patient selection in UAS and must be performed and recorded in a systematic manner.
- Modifications must be made to surgical techniques used in adults in order to account for challenges unique to children with DS, including patient positioning, incision planning, and postoperative care.
- Device programming is essential for ensuring optimal outcomes. Modification must be made to existing programming protocols used in adults.

DISCLOSURE

No conflicts of interest. This study was not funded.

REFERENCES

1. Shott SR. Down syndrome: common otolaryngologic manifestations. Am J Med Genet C Semin Med Genet 2006;142c(3):131–40.
2. Horne RS, Wijayaratne P, Nixon GM, et al. Sleep and sleep disordered breathing in children with down syndrome: Effects on behaviour, neurocognition and the cardiovascular system. Sleep Med Rev 2019;44:1–11.
3. Menzies B, Teng A, Burns M, et al. Neurocognitive outcomes of children with sleep disordered breathing: A systematic review with meta-analysis. Sleep Med Rev 2022;63:101629.
4. Mitchell RB, Archer SM, Ishman SL, et al. Clinical Practice Guideline: Tonsillectomy in Children (Update). Otolaryngol Head Neck Surg 2019;160(1_suppl): S1–42.
5. Ingram DG, Ruiz AG, Gao D, et al. Success of Tonsillectomy for Obstructive Sleep Apnea in Children With Down Syndrome. J Clin Sleep Med 2017;13(8): 975–80.
6. Nation J, Brigger M. The Efficacy of Adenotonsillectomy for Obstructive Sleep Apnea in Children with Down Syndrome: A Systematic Review. Otolaryngol Head Neck Surg 2017;157(3):401–8.
7. Nehme J, LaBerge R, Pothos M, et al. Treatment and persistence/recurrence of sleep-disordered breathing in children with Down syndrome. Pediatr Pulmonol 2019;54(8):1291–6.
8. Tauman R, Gulliver TE, Krishna J, et al. Persistence of obstructive sleep apnea syndrome in children after adenotonsillectomy. J Pediatr 2006;149(6):803–8.
9. Hyzer JM, Milczuk HA, Macarthur CJ, et al. Drug-Induced Sleep Endoscopy Findings in Children With Obstructive Sleep Apnea With vs Without Obesity or Down Syndrome. JAMA Otolaryngol Head Neck Surg 2021;147(2):175–81.
10. Trucco F, Chatwin M, Semple T, et al. Sleep disordered breathing and ventilatory support in children with Down syndrome. Pediatr Pulmonol 2018;53(10):1414–21.
11. Woodson BT, Soose RJ, Gillespie MB, et al. Three-Year Outcomes of Cranial Nerve Stimulation for Obstructive Sleep Apnea: The STAR Trial. Otolaryngol Head Neck Surg 2016;154(1):181–8.
12. Yu PK, Stenerson M, Ishman SL, et al. Evaluation of Upper Airway Stimulation for Adolescents With Down Syndrome and Obstructive Sleep Apnea. JAMA Otolaryngol Head Neck Surg 2022;148(6):522–8.
13. Inspire Medical Systems, Inc. Announces FDA Approval for Pediatric Patients with Down Syndrome. Inspire Medical Systems. 2023. Available at: https://investors.inspiresleep.com/investors/press-releases/press-release-details/2023/Inspire-Medical-Systems-Inc.-Announces-FDA-Approval-for-Pediatric-Patients-with-Down-Syndrome/default.aspx.
14. Van de Heyning PH, Badr MS, Baskin JZ, et al. Implanted upper airway stimulation device for obstructive sleep apnea. Laryngoscope 2012;122(7):1626–33.
15. Vanderveken OM, Maurer JT, Hohenhorst W, et al. Evaluation of drug-induced sleep endoscopy as a patient selection tool for implanted upper airway stimulation for obstructive sleep apnea. J Clin Sleep Med 2013;9(5):433–8.
16. Huyett P, Kent DT, D'Agostino MA, et al. Drug-Induced Sleep Endoscopy and Hypoglossal Nerve Stimulation Outcomes: A Multicenter Cohort Study. Laryngoscope 2021;131(7):1676–82.

17. Goding GS Jr, Tesfayesus W, Kezirian EJ. Hypoglossal nerve stimulation and airway changes under fluoroscopy. Otolaryngol Head Neck Surg 2012;146(6): 1017–22.
18. Baldassari CM, Lam DJ, Ishman SL, et al. Expert Consensus Statement: Pediatric Drug-Induced Sleep Endoscopy. Otolaryngol Head Neck Surg 2021;165(4): 578–91.
19. Heiser C, Thaler E, Boon M, et al. Updates of operative techniques for upper airway stimulation. Laryngoscope 2016;126(Suppl 7):S12–6.
20. Bowe SN, Diercks GR, Hartnick CJ. Modified surgical approach to hypoglossal nerve stimulator implantation in the pediatric population. Laryngoscope 2018; 128(6):1490–2.
21. Sagalow ES, Rodin J, Estephan L, et al. Two-Incision Approach for Hypoglossal Nerve Stimulator Placement: A Single Institution Assessment. Laryngoscope 2022;132(8):1687–91.
22. Kent DT, Chio EG, Weiner JS, et al. A Noninferiority Analysis of 3- vs 2-Incision Techniques for Hypoglossal Nerve Stimulator Implantation. Otolaryngol Head Neck Surg 2022;167(1):197–202.
23. Sadove AM, van Aalst JA. Congenital and acquired pediatric breast anomalies: a review of 20 years' experience. Plast Reconstr Surg 2005;115(4):1039–50.
24. Morse E, Dodhia S, Suurna M. Upper Airway Stimulation in Female Patients: Safety and Efficacy of a Novel Lateral Approach. Otolaryngol Head Neck Surg 2023. https://doi.org/10.1002/ohn.225.
25. McGuire BE, Defrin R. Pain perception in people with Down syndrome: a synthesis of clinical and experimental research. Front Behav Neurosci 2015;9:194.
26. Soose RJ, Faber K, Greenberg H, et al. Post-implant care pathway: lessons learned and recommendations after 5 years of clinical implementation of hypoglossal nerve stimulation therapy. Sleep 2021;44(Supplement_1):S4–10.

Neurostimulation for Obstructive Sleep Apnea

Maria V. Suurna, MD*, Mia Klasner, FNP-BC, MSN

KEYWORDS

- Neurostimulation • Obstructive sleep apnea • Hypoglossal nerve stimulation
- Sleep apnea treatment • Alternative to CPAP treatment • Sleep disordered breathing

KEY POINTS

- Obstructive sleep apnea (OSA) is a heterogeneous disorder characterized by symptomatic, repeated airway collapse during sleep.
- Neurostimulation of hypoglossal nerve has emerged as an effective treatment option of OSA.
- Ongoing research and technological developments continue to advance the therapy to deliver personalized and efficient treatment to patients with OSA.

INTRODUCTION

Obstructive sleep apnea (OSA) is a heterogeneous disorder characterized by symptomatic, repeated airway collapse during sleep. Patients with untreated sleep apnea often seek treatment for complaints of excessive snoring, daytime sleepiness, and poor sleep quality.[1] Positive airway pressure (PAP) is often the first-line treatment for patients with symptomatic disease.[2] However, due to many competing factors, such as poor PAP tolerance and compliance, long-term treatment is often ineffective.[3] In the past decade, hypoglossal nerve stimulation therapy (HNS) has evolved as an effective alternative treatment option for patients with moderate-to-severe OSA.

This treatment concept is not new and the stimulation of the hypoglossal nerve to allow for airway expansion during sleep has been under investigation in humans since 1990. Patients with OSA have underlying upper airway compromise that predisposes them to airway collapse during sleep. Within the airway, the genioglossus muscle is the predominant factor in maintaining a dilated upper airway and contributes to tongue protrusion. Retroglossal airway opening can be achieved by engaging genioglossus muscle through stimulation of the hypoglossal nerve. In 1997, the study results demonstrated significant improvements in ventilation with stimulation of the hypoglossal

Department of Otolaryngology–Head and Neck Surgery, University of Miami Miller School of Medicine, University of Miami Health System, 1120 Northwest 14th Street, 5th Floor, Miami, FL 33136, USA
* Corresponding author.
E-mail address: maria.suurna@miami.edu

Otolaryngol Clin N Am 57 (2024) 457–465
https://doi.org/10.1016/j.otc.2024.02.003
oto.theclinics.com

nerve.[4] In 2001, a 2 center trial demonstrated reduction of the number of obstructive events during sleep with hypoglossal nerve stimulation.[5] In 2014, the multicenter Stimulation Therapy for Apnea Reduction (STAR) trial published results that led to FDA approval for HNS.[6] This therapy became available to patients as an effective treatment option for OSA in the United States for those patients who are intolerant to or cannot benefit from traditional PAP therapy. Since initial approval, HNS availability has become more expansive as evolving FDA criteria have begun to include more patients as surgical candidates.

NERVE ANATOMY

To fully comprehend the mechanism of HNS, it is important to have a clear understanding of the anatomy of the targeted nerve. The hypoglossal nerve is a cranial nerve 12 (CNXII) with pure somatic motor function, which is responsible for speaking, swallowing, and maintaining an open oropharyngeal airway. The HNS is responsible, during sleep, for activating the upper airway muscles to allow for airway stabilization and opening. This opening occurs at multiple points within the retropalatal, retroglossal, and retroepiglottic airway space.[7]

The hypoglossal nerve emanates from the hypoglossal nucleus in the medulla oblongata and exits the brainstem via the anterolateral sulcus. It subsequently travels through the hypoglossal canal to exit the cranial vault, descending vertically in the retrostyloid space. It then turns anteriorly and courses laterally over the external carotid artery. Once emerging from this space, it runs deep to the submandibular gland, the posterior belly of the digastric muscle, the mylohyoid muscle, and superficial to the hyoglossus (HG) muscle.

The nerve is divided into medial and lateral branches that can be identified as it runs over the HG muscle. The extrinsic muscles of the tongue that are innervated by the medial division of CNXII include the genioglossus horizontal (GGh) and the genioglossus oblique (GGo) muscles. It is important to note that the GGh muscle facilitates forward tongue movement, while the GGo muscle controls downward tongue movement. The styloglossus (SG) and HG muscles are innervated by the lateral division of CNXII and are also considered to be extrinsic muscles. The SG muscle allows for retraction and elevation of the tongue, while the HG muscle allows for retraction and depression of the tongue.[8]

CNXII innervates 5 separate intrinsic muscles, which each serve their own function to support tongue movement. The inferior longitudinal medial (m-IL) muscle, transverse (T) muscle, and vertical (V) muscle are all innervated by the medial division of CNXII. The m-IL muscle works to shorten the tongue and curl the tip inferiorly; the T muscle narrows the tongue; and the V muscle flattens the tongue. The final 2 intrinsic muscles are innervated by the lateral division on CNXII. The superior longitudinal shortens the tongue and curls the tip superiorly. Finally, the inferior longitudinal lateral muscle shortens the tongue and curls the tip inferiorly.[8]

The hypoglossal nerve is consistently accompanied by nerve fibers from C1/C2 roots. C1/C2 nerve fibers travel with the hypoglossal nerve and eventually exit at the inferior portion of the nerve. At this point, they innervate the geniohyoid muscle and join ansa cervicalis to innervate the infrahyoid strap muscles. The location and course of these fibers in relation to the hypoglossal nerve varies patient to patient. This variability will influence the ability to include or exclude them into the stimulation cuff. While not a surgical requirement for therapy efficacy, incorporating C1/C2 fibers in the stimulation cuff will result in contraction of the geniohyoid muscle leading to elevation and movement of the hyoid bone anteriorly.[9] Although still somewhat controversial as to the benefits of including C1/C2 in the cuff, the consensus remains that inclusion of C1/2 has the potential to benefit in outcomes of HNS.

Preoperative Evaluation

Preoperative evaluation is used to identify those patients that will benefit most from therapeutic intervention with HNS. Standard baseline evaluation should include a thorough review of the patient's sleep history to confirm moderate-to-severe OSA and assess for comorbid sleep disorders, medical/surgical history, and physical assessment including drug-induced sleep endoscopy (DISE).[10] HNS has been indicated for patients with moderate-to-severe OSA with an apnea–hypopnea index (AHI) between 15 and 65 and a BMI up to 32 kg/m^2. Additional therapy indication parameters include central/mixed apnea events comprising less than 25% of the total AHI on a sleep study and absence of complete concentric palatal/velopharyngeal collapse on DISE.[6] However, recently FDA indications for the HNS thearpy utilizing device manufactured by Inspire Medical have been expanded to an AHI ranging from 15 to 100 and a BMI up to 40 kg/m^2. Based on FDA labeling, HNS is suitable for patients if they have failed or are unable to tolerate PAP therapy. PAP therapy is still considered to be the first-line treatment of OSA and should not be bypassed as a treatment option in patients considering HNS. Nonetheless, based on published literature, around 30% to 40% of patients are nonadherent with PAP therapy.[3] Therefore, despite advances in PAP therapy (eg, mask improvements, smaller systems, and quieter devices), patients continue to require alternative options for treatment of OSA.

DISE is currently used to assess the patient's nature of airway obstruction during sleep prior to implantation of the HNS. DISE allows for real-time examination of the pattern of upper airway collapse. The previous studies have indicated that patients who exhibited complete concentric palatal collapse were less likely to achieve surgical success with HNS.[11] Depending on the outcome of the DISE examination, HNS can be considered in the qualifying patient. Some patients may benefit from other surgical interventions including uvulopalatopharyngoplasty (UPPP) or tonsillectomy. These secondary options should be presented and considered by the patient prior to pursuing HNS as recommended by the FDA.

Current guidelines for the Inspire device specify parameters for patients undergoing MRI to not expose the device to a power greater than 1.5 T. This is a critical consideration in patients who have anticipated needs of future MRIs.

Surgical Technique

At present, the most utilized and widely available hypoglossal nerve stimulation device is manufactured by Inspire Medical Systems. The system consists of an implantable pulse generator (IPG) implanted in the infraclavicular area, a neurostimulation lead with a cuff placed on the medial fibers of the hypoglossal nerve, and a respiratory sensor lead located in the second or third intercostal space.[12–14] Intraoperatively, it is imperative that proper identification of the medial and lateral nerve fibers is achieved prior to cuff placement. This detection is accomplished by utilizing the nerve integrity monitoring (NIM) system.

The patient is initially placed supine with the head slightly extended prior to anesthesia. After induction of general anesthesia, the airway is secured with either a transoral or transnasal endotracheal tube, the bed is then rotated 180° with the head of the bed opposite the anesthesiology machine. With transoral intubation, the endotracheal tube is secured on the left side of the oral cavity to reduce interference with the tongue and surgical space assuming the patient is undergoing right-sided surgery. It is imperative to note that muscle relaxant or paralytic agents should not be used during the procedure as it can impair the ability to properly monitor the nerve function.

On the ipsilateral side of the implant, single-use Prass Paired Electromyography (EMG) 18-mm needle electrodes are inserted into the genioglossus (GG) muscle through the floor of the mouth slightly off midline and submucosally into the HG/SG muscles running along the ventral side of the lateral tongue approximately 5 cm from the tip of the tongue. A proper placement and use of the EMG electrodes aids in isolating out any nerve fibers that may cause tongue retraction. The area from the edge of the mandible down to the mid-chest is then prepped using a betadine solution. The area is then draped combining Ioban from the edge of the mandible, extending down the surgical field and a clear drape placed from the superior edge of the mandible over the mouth and head to allow for direct visualization of the tongue intraoperatively while maintaining sterility.

A 3 to 5 cm incision is placed in the patient's neck crease or parallel to the relaxed skin tension lines approximately 1 to 2 cm below the mandible from the anterior border of the submandibular gland extending toward midline. Once the platysma muscle is divided, the anterior border of the submandibular gland is identified. The gland is retracted posteriorly, and dissection is carried further toward the digastric muscle tendon which is retracted inferiorly. Then, the posterior border of the mylohyoid muscle is retracted anteriorly to allow for clear visualization of the hypoglossal nerve. Typically, the ranine vein can be visualized running on top of the nerve. Usually, this vein can be preserved and dissected away from the nerve; however, in occasional cases, vein ligation is necessary for adequate nerve exposure.

Once the hypoglossal nerve has been identified, distal dissection of the nerve is performed to identify medial branches of the nerve. A small vasa nervorum often helps identify the break point between lateral and medial branches of the nerve. Often, C1/C2 nerve fibers can be seen coursing along the inferior edge of the nerve. Attempt should be made to include these fibers in the stimulation cuff. Once the breaking point is identified, a bipolar nerve stimulation probe is used to confirm the function of the identified fibers based on EMG responses on the NIM at 0.1 to 0.3 V. When lateral nerve branches are stimulated, polyphasic EMG response is seen on the SG/HG channel. Owing to the risk of including retractor branches in the cuff, nerve stimulation should be performed on the superior edge of the medial division to ensure no unwanted branches are included. Care should be taken to exclude these identified branches from the stimulation cuff. When medial nerve branches are stimulated, monophasic response is seen on the GG channel. The stimulation cuff is then wrapped around the isolated medical branches of the nerve. The cuff is then flushed with saline to remove any air between the cuff and the nerve. The lead is anchored to the digastric tendon using a 3-0 silk suture.

For placement of the IPG and respiratory lead, a 4 to 5 cm transverse chest incision is placed in the area above the second or third intercostal space. Dissection is carried down to the pectoralis major muscle. An inferior pocket for IPG is created superficial to the muscle fascia. Pectoralis major muscle fibers are separated using blunt dissection at the level of the second or third intercostal space. With dissection in the intercostal space, external intercostal muscle fibers are identified, the fibers are separated to expose the underlying internal intercostal muscle. The tip of the respiratory sensor lead is placed in the space between internal and external intercostal muscles directed toward the axilla. The proximal lead anchor is secured to the external intercostal muscle, and the distal lead anchor is secured to the pectoralis muscle.

The stimulation lead is tunneled from the submandibular incision toward the IPG pocket in the subplatysmal plane and above the clavicle. The stimulation and respiratory leads are connected and secured to the IPG using preset screws. Any excess lead wire is then coiled and placed deep into the pocket posterior to the IPG. Using a 2-0 silk suture, the IPG is secured to the pectoralis major fascia.

Once the IPG is secured, the system is interrogated to confirm proper function. The telemetry wand is brought into the sterile field using a sterile covering and placed on the skin above the IPG. The respiratory sensor wave is checked for proper detection of inspiration and expiration. In the event, a clear wave pattern is not identified, and the respiratory sensor placement should be explored and modified if necessary. The stimulation lead function is then checked via direct visualization of tongue motion in response to device activation. The tongue motion and EMG signals are analyzed utilizing bipolar and unipolar settings at various voltages.[15] Suitable tongue motion and proper placement of the stimulation cuff on the nerve can be characterized as unrestricted forward tongue protrusion. Improper or mixed activation can be identified by visualizing retraction of the tongue to the ipsilateral side of the implant and having polyphasic activity in SG/HG EMG channel. If this is seen, reexploration and repositioning of the stimulation cuff needs to be performed to exclude any late retractor branches. Once comprehensive electrical testing of the implant is complete, the wounds are irrigated, and a multilayer closure is performed for all incisions. Following the incision closure steri strips and pressure dressing are placed over the incisions.

Postoperative Care

Prior to surgery, patients undergoing implantation of HNS device should be counseled on the risks of surgery, recovery process, and postsurgical expectations. Though extremely rare, procedure-related adverse events can occur. Risks can include bleeding, infection, hematoma or seroma, injury or weakness to the hypoglossal or marginal mandibular nerves, and pneumothorax.[9] Prior to discharge, all patients need an upright chest radiograph and lateral neck radiograph. This aids in documentation of baseline device position, proper electrode placement, and ruling out pneumothorax. Typically, patients can be discharged home the same day of surgery based on institutional recovery room protocols. Patients usually do not require opioid medications for pain management and can often use acetaminophen and/or ibuprofen for pain relief. If relevant, patients can restart anticoagulation medications 24 hours after surgery. During the discharge process, the patient is educated regarding proper incision care and postoperative activity restrictions. During the first 2 weeks postoperatively, the patient is instructed to avoid strenuous activity and restrict movement of the arm and shoulder on the surgical side.

The initial follow-up postoperative visits occur at 1 week and again at 4 to 6 weeks from the date of implantation. At the 1 week appointment, the incision is checked for proper healing and the patient is assessed for any postoperative adverse events. Device activation and programming occur at the 4 to 6 week visit. Once the device is activated, proper system function is verified including proper response of the respiratory sensor. Frequently, therapy is initiated with the default stimulation settings. These settings correspond to bipolar electrode configuration [+-+], pulse width 90 μs, and rate 33 Hz.[10] The functional threshold, defined as the lowest amplitude at which tongue protrusion passes the mandibular incisors, is then established. Initial amplitude is usually set at the level of the functional threshold. The device is programmed to have a patient control range of ten 0.1 V increments starting one increment below the functional threshold.[10]

Following device activation, patients start therapy nightly by turning it on with the remote control before going to bed. The therapy start delay time and pause time are set based on the patient's preferences and sleep habits, with default settings of a 30 minute start delay and 15 minute pause. The patient is then instructed on use of the remote control and how to self-titrate the device. Self-titration allows patients to gradually increase the stimulation level weekly to achieve optimal therapy comfort and symptom improvement. It is important to instruct patients to avoid stimulation past their therapy comfort level.

In certain circumstances, there is indication to delay therapy activation or adjust settings beyond the default stimulation settings. If indicated by suboptimal tongue motion in the bipolar settings, therapy can be initiated in unipolar settings [-o-; o-o;—]. In cases when neuropraxia or tongue weakness is noted, therapy activation should be delayed until full recovery of tongue function is achieved.

After 1 to 2 months of therapy use, patients are scheduled for follow-up to assess subjective benefits of the therapy. During this appointment, further testing can be arranged to assess the objective effectiveness of therapy. In-laboratory polysomnography is traditionally used to fine-tune and further titrate stimulation for optimal therapy outcomes. However, home sleep apnea testing (HSAT) has been increasingly used to assess therapy effectiveness at the patient's self-optimized settings. If the HSAT confirms adequate control of sleep apnea, the patient is instructed to continue the therapy use at the optimized therapy settings.

In cases with inadequate objective and/or subjective response, in-office therapy adjustments or in-laboratory therapy optimization should be considered. In-office advanced programming can be performed with direct airway visualization with a laryngoscope. With direct visualization of the airway, various combinations of the device settings such as amplitude, pulse width, rate, and electrode configuration can be systematically analyzed and modified based on the observed airway response to the stimulation.

Once therapy effectiveness is established, the patients are instructed to continue therapy use every night and follow-up in 6 to 12 months for device check and adjustment if necessary. At that time, another HSAT can be performed to further evaluate therapy efficacy. During follow-up visits, therapy adherence is checked utilizing online device resources. Technology allows for downloading of therapy compliance data directly from the remote or via the Bluetooth connection to the device phone application. Timely intervention is essential if poor therapy adherence is recognized to assure best therapy outcomes. Once adequate compliance and positive results have been established, the patient should transition to long-term management. Even though device battery longevity is estimated to be 10+ years, patients should still be followed annually. At this visit, the device should be checked, compliance data reviewed, clinical assessment performed, and therapy modified if needed to maintain therapeutic outcomes. Patients who are struggling with therapy adherence, have persistent symptoms, or elevated AHI with therapy on, should be considered for multimodality therapy. These interventions can include weight loss, positional therapy, additional surgical interventions, oral appliance therapy, or other treatments to further improve the effectiveness of HNS and reduce symptomatic burden of OSA.[16]

Clinical Evidence

Effectiveness of HNS on humans for management of OSA was demonstrated by the outcomes from the STAR trial. This study led to FDA approval of the device manufactured by Inspire Medical. During a 12 month period, the study measured polysomnographic and quality of life indicators as it related to device safety and effectiveness.[6] The trial consisted of 126 participants with an AHI of 20 to 50, a central/mixed apnea index less than 25%, no evidence of tonsillar hypertrophy, BMI less than 32 kg/m^2, and displayed no evidence of complete concentric collapse on DISE. A positive response to therapy qualified as a decrease in AHI of 50% and under 20 events per hour. Secondary measures were tested to evaluate quality-of- life improvement utilizing Epworth Sleepiness Scale (ESS) and Funcrional Outcomes of Sleep Questionnaire (FOSQ). Results demonstrated 68% reduction in AHI with the therapy use from a median of 29.3 preoperatively to a median of 9 postoperatively. Additional results demonstrated improvements in ESS and FOSQ scores. Within the study, the overall rate of serious adverse events was 2%, supporting the notion of relative therapy safety.[6] Participants of the STAR trial continued to be reassessed at 18, 24, 36, 48, and 60 months. Follow-up outcomes continue to demonstrate long-term therapy effectiveness.[17–20]

The ongoing ADHERE Registry is a prospective observational study that aims to deepen the evaluation of real-world outcomes to the HNS. The goal of this registry is to assess polysomnographic changes, quality-of-life improvement, and surgical outcomes in patients undergoing HNS outside of a clinical trial environment. Data suggest continued reduction in AHI with baseline median AHI of 32.8 decreasing to 6.3 and 9.5 at the 6 and 12 month follow up, respectively.[21] Further data showed a significant reduction in ESS; at the baseline visit, median ESS was 11 and subsequently decreased to 6.0 at the 12 month visit. During this analysis, female gender and reduced BMI were shown to be predictors of good response.[21] All in all, 90% of patients who participated in the ADHERE registry preferred HNS over CPAP therapy.[22] Patients with higher BMI in ADHERE were also shown to benefit from HNS. Finally, it was also demonstrated that therapy comfort is important in assuring long-term compliance and better outcomes.[23] These results suggest that with focused patient selection, proper adherence, and close follow-up, HNS is an effective, safe, and suitable alternative to traditional OSA treatments.

In comparison to other surgical alternatives, HNS demonstrated better results in reducing AHI in patients with OSA. In a study that compared UPPP to HNS, patients who underwent HNS had a mean AHI decrease from 38.9 to 4.5, while patients who underwent UPPP had mean AHI decrease from 40.3 to 28.8.[24] Huntley and colleagues similarly demonstrated a substantially greater decrease in AHI severity within the HNS group compared to the traditional upper airway surgery group, further supporting improved efficacy of HNS for OSA management. It is worth mentioning that the differences in ESS scores were negligible when comparing the 2 groups.[25]

Evolving Technology

With the notable advances provided by the HNS, an increasing number of medical device companies are seeking to manufacture and offer devices to treat OSA. The Genio system manufactured by Nyxoah is an implantable neurostimulation device, which is designed to activate genioglossus muscle bilaterally. This system utilizes a small implanted neurostimulator and is activated by an external piece applied nightly by the patient. Through a single incision, the device is positioned over the genioglossus muscles and delivers stimulation to the bilateral hypoglossal nerve branches. The implanted piece is activated by an external unit which generates cyclical energy pulses, giving the patient's rest periods between impulses and therefore omits the need for a respiratory sensor. Unlike other devices, this system may be perceived as less invasive since it involves only one incision in the submental region and requires the implantation of only one component, foregoing the need for a respiratory sensor or IPG. The initial study results with Nyxoah revealed improvements in AHI, ESS scores, and quality of life.[26]

The Aura6000 by LivaNova is another emerging technology. This device directly targets the hypoglossal nerve but does not require dissection of the nerve to exclude retractor branches. Instead, this process includes a 6 electrode cuff placed around the nerve allowing for stimulation of many of the tongue muscles, which leads to tongue protrusion and pharyngeal wall opening. Candidacy evaluation for this therapy does not require DISE before implantation, as complete concentric collapse is not a contraindication for this therapy. The stimulation lead for Aura6000 is connected to a pulse generator which is placed subcutaneously in the infraclavicular region of the chest and activated using an external recharging remote control. This device does not include a respiratory sensor and the therapy operates on a duty cycle.[27]

Technological developments, combined with ongoing research efforts, underscore the growing interest and potential of HNS in the realm of OSA management and personalized patient care. As medical industry strives to contribute to this evolving field, the future holds promising possibilities for the continual improvement and accessibility of the HNS as an effective solution for individuals with OSA.

DISCLOSURE

M.V. Suurna: Inspire Medical - Consultant; Nyxoah - Consultant, clinical trial site primary investigator; Livanova -clinical trial site primary investigator.

REFERENCES

1. Gambino F, Zammuto MM, Virzì A, et al. Treatment options in obstructive sleep apnea. Intern Emerg Med 2022;17(4):971–8.
2. Sullivan CE, Issa FG, Berthon-Jones M, et al. Reversal of obstructive sleep apnoea by continuous positive airway pressure applied through the nares. Lancet 1981;1:862.
3. Rotenberg BW, Murariu D, Pang KP. Trends in CPAP adherence over twenty years of data collection: a flattened curve. J Otolaryngol Head Neck Surg 2016;45:43.
4. Eisele DW, Smith PL, Alam DS, et al. Direct hypoglossal nerve stimulation in obstructive sleep apnea. Arch Otolaryngol Head Neck Surg 1997;123(1):57–61.
5. Schwartz AR, Bennett ML, Smith PL, et al. Therapeutic electrical stimulation of the hypoglossal nerve in obstructive sleep apnea. Arch Otolaryngol Head Neck Surg 2001;127(10):1216–23.
6. Strollo PJ, Soose RJ, Maurer JT, et al. Upper-airway stimulation for obstructive sleep apnea. N Engl J Med 2014;370(2):139–49.
7. Safiruddin F, Vanderveken OM, de Vries N, et al. Effect of upper-airway stimulation for obstructive sleep apnoea on airway dimensions. Eur Respir J 2015;45(1):129–38.
8. Mu L, Sanders I. Human tongue neuroanatomy: nerve supply and motor endplates. Clin Anat 2010;23(7):777–91.
9. Suurna MV. Hypoglossal nerve stimulation for adult patients with obstructive sleep apnea. In: Post T, editor. Waltham, Mass: UpToDate; 2023. www.uptodate.com. [Accessed 3 January 2023].
10. Strollo PJ Jr, Gillespie MB, Soose RJ, et al. Upper airway stimulation for obstructive sleep apnea: durability of the treatment effect at 18 months. Sleep 2015;38(10):1593–8.
11. Vanderveken OM, Maurer JT, Hohenhorst W, et al. Evaluation of drug-induced sleep endoscopy as a patient selection tool for implanted upper airway stimulation for obstructive sleep apnea. J Clin Sleep Med 2013;9(5):433–8.
12. Maurer JT, Van de Heyning P, Lin HS, et al. Operative technique of upper airway stimulation: an implantable treatment of obstructive sleep apnea. Operat Tech Otolaryngol Head Neck Surg 2012;23(3):227–33.

13. Heiser C, Thaler E, Boon M, et al. Updates of operative techniques for upper airway stimulation: operative techniques for UAS. Laryngoscope 2016;126:S12–6.
14. Kent DT, Weiner JS, Chio EG, et al. Hypoglossal nerve stimulator implantation via a 2-incision technique. Oper Tech Otolayngol Head Neck Surg 2020;31(3): e35–42.
15. Sturm JJ, Lee CH, Modik O, et al. Intraoperative identification of mixed activation profiles during hypoglossal nerve stimulation. J Clin Sleep Med 2020;16(10): 1769–74.
16. Olson MD, Junna MR. Hypoglossal nerve stimulation therapy for the treatment of obstructive sleep apnea. Neurotherapeutics 2021;18:91–9.
17. Soose RJ, Woodson BT, Gillespie MB, et al. Upper airway stimulation for obstructive sleep apnea: self-reported outcomes at 24 months. J Clin Sleep Med 2016; 12(1):43–8.
18. Woodson BT, Soose RJ, Gillespie MB, et al. Three-year outcomes of cranial nerve stimulation for obstructive sleep apnea: the star trial. Otolaryng Head Neck 2016; 154(1):181–8.
19. Gillespie MB, Soose RJ, Woodson BT, et al. Upper airway stimulation for obstructive sleep apnea: patient-reported outcomes after 48 months of follow-up. Otolaryng Head Neck 2017;156(4):765–71.
20. Woodson BT, Strohl KP, Soose RJ, et al. Upper airway stimulation for obstructive sleep apnea: 5-year outcomes. Otolaryngol Head Neck Surg 2018;159(1): 194–202.
21. Thaler E, Schwab R, Maurer J, et al. Results of the ADHERE upper airway stimulation registry and predictors of therapy efficacy. Laryngoscope 2020;130(5): 1333–8.
22. Boon M, Huntley C, Steffen A, et al, ADHERE Registry Investigators. Upper airway stimulation for obstructive sleep apnea: results from the ADHERE registry. Otolaryngology-Head Neck Surg (Tokyo) 2018;159:379–85.
23. Suurna MV, Steffen A, Boon M, et al, ADHERE Registry Investigators. Impact of body mass index and discomfort on upper airway stimulation: ADHERE registry 2020 update. Laryngoscope 2021;131(11):2616–24.
24. Shah J, Russell JO, Waters T, et al. Uvulopalatopharyngoplasty vs CN XII stimulation for treatment of obstructive sleep apnea: A single institution experience. Am J Otolaryngol 2018;39(3):266–70.
25. Huntley C, Boon M, Tschopp S, et al. Comparison of traditional upper airway surgery and upper airway stimulation for obstructive sleep apnea. Ann Otol Rhinol Laryngol 2021;130(4):370–6.
26. Eastwood PR, Barnes M, MacKay SG, et al. Bilateral hypoglossal nerve stimulation for treatment of adult obstructive sleep apnoea. Eur Respir J 2020;55(1): 1901320.
27. Mwenge GB, Rombaux P, Dury M, et al. Targeted hypoglossal neurostimulation for obstructive sleep apnoea: a 1-year pilot study. Eur Respir J 2013;41(2):360–7.

Sex Differences in Obstructive Sleep Apnea Including Pregnancy and Response to Treatment

Taylor S. Erickson, MD[a], Megan L. Durr, MD[b,*]

KEYWORDS

• Pregnancy • Sex differences • Women • Treatment

KEY POINTS

- Obstructive sleep apnea (OSA) is more common in men than women, but women may present with more atypical symptoms, which can contribute to underdiagnosis.
- The primary treatment algorithm of OSA is the same for men and women, yet treatment effectiveness may vary between these 2 populations.
- OSA prevalence during mid-to-late pregnancy is around 15% and is associated with adverse maternal and fetal outcomes.
- Although surgical treatment in pregnancy is generally not feasible, otolaryngologists can still play a role in comanaging OSA in pregnancy.

INTRODUCTION

Obstructive sleep apnea (OSA) is a widespread sleep disorder that affects all populations; however, the presentation and clinical manifestations of the condition often exhibit distinct differences between men and women. While both sexes may experience similar disruptions in breathing patterns during sleep, a growing body of research suggests that men and women may manifest varying symptoms, risk factors, and treatment outcomes related to sleep apnea. OSA in pregnancy poses unique diagnostic and therapeutic challenges given the relative dearth of literature on this topic as well as some of the treatment considerations unique to this patient population. The current article reviews the variances in prevalence, diagnosis, and treatment of

[a] Department of Otolaryngology–Head & Neck Surgery, University of California, San Francisco, 2233 Post Street, San Francisco, CA 94115, USA; [b] Department of Otolaryngology–Head & Neck Surgery, University of California, San Francisco, 1001 Potrero Avenue, #3A30, San Francisco, CA 94110, USA
* Corresponding author.
E-mail address: Megan.Durr@ucsf.edu

Otolaryngol Clin N Am 57 (2024) 467–480
https://doi.org/10.1016/j.otc.2024.02.001

OSA between male and female individuals, including a review of special considerations within the pregnant population.

Prevalence

OSA is more common in men than women with an estimated prevalence ranging from 13% to 33% in adult men and 6% to 19% in adult women[1] corresponding to an approximate 2:1 ratio.[2] Previously proposed explanations for such a discrepancy include increased sex differences in body fat distribution, specifically increased upper airway fat distribution in men,[3] as well as differences in pharyngeal anatomy and function. Specifically, upper airway length (distance between hard palate and the superior posterior hyoid bone) is longer in men than in women, which correlates with greater susceptibility to airway collapse and more severe OSA.[4,5]

Differences in Presentation

It has been increasingly acknowledged that women may have more atypical presentations than men leading to a relative underdiagnosis of OSA in women.[2] Studies have shown that the male OSA predominance seen in epidemiologic studies is likely even more noteworthy in the clinical setting with estimates of the male-to-female ratio being as high as 8 to 10:1.

Women more commonly report nonspecific symptoms such as fatigue, insomnia, tension, and use of sedatives[3,6–8] and are more commonly misdiagnosed with depression.[9] These symptoms differ from those more historically associated with OSA, including snoring, gasping, and apneic episodes with which men commonly present.[10,11] Additional studies have suggested that women may be underdiagnosed due to circumstances related to sociocultural factors.[12,13] Women are less likely to present to clinic while accompanied by their bed partners as compared to men. This leads to difficulty detecting nocturnal symptoms and likely lowers diagnostic ability.[14] In addition to anatomic differences, variations in how OSA presents and the potential for underdiagnosis in women could account for some of the aforementioned disparities in prevalence.

Obstructive Sleep Apnea and Menopause

There appears to be a hormonal effect on OSA. There is no observed sex difference in OSA prevalence in the pediatric population followed by increased risk for males in the middle age group. Then, OSA prevalence becomes equivalent again for elderly men and women.[12]

There is an increased prevalence of OSA in female patients after menopause.[15,16] Menopause is characterized by the gradual, steady decline in progesterone and estrogen levels often accompanied by sleep disturbances, and women with sleep apnea are reported to have lower levels of circulating estrogen and progesterone.[17] Progesterone and estrogen have been shown to have stimulatory effect on ventilation drive and also on expanding the upper airway tract.[18] Additionally, changes in sex hormones after menopause increase fat distribution in the abdomen and are associated with an increased neck circumference, which also increases the risk of apnea.[19] The activity of the genioglossus muscle, an important pharyngeal dilator, has been shown to lower after menopause and may increase with hormone replacement therapy (HRT).[18]

Obesity

Obesity defined as BMI $\geq$ 30 kg/m^2 has been widely recognized as having a strong connection with OSA in both male and female individuals.[20] Interestingly, despite a higher prevalence of obesity in females than males,[21] men have higher rates of OSA. Additionally, when matched for BMI, men have been shown to demonstrate more severe OSA as compared to their female counterparts, and as BMI increases, the severity of OSA increases disproportionally in male as compared to female population.[22–24] This may be related to the more gynecoid fat distribution in women versus central fat distribution in men. Central fat distribution has been shown to be more related to development of OSA,[25] so obese men may be more susceptible to developing OSA than their female counterparts. Researchers have suggested that men also experience a disproportionate increase in upper airway collapsibility with additional weight gain, though this remains an area for further investigation.[22]

TREATMENT DIFFERENCES

Weight Loss

Given the known association between obesity and OSA, weight loss has been well studied as an effective treatment for OSA. Interestingly, weight loss in patients with OSA has been shown to be more successful in men than in women as a treatment.[14,26] Such findings may be attributed to women having a more anatomically stable upper airway, making it less susceptible to weight-related changes as previously discussed. Bariatric surgery has proven to be an effective OSA treatment due to its ability to provide a sustainable, long-term solution for weight loss.[27] The majority of studies examining how bariatric surgery impacts the severity of OSA have not specified sex-specific differences in efficacy. Among the studies that have explored this aspect, no distinctions in effectiveness between men and women have been observed.[28]

Continuous Positive Airway Pressure

Continuous positive airway pressure (CPAP) represents the cornerstone of OSA therapy through its ability to dilate the upper airway. The data on CPAP compliance and efficacy as a treatment for OSA between men and women are conflicting. Studies have demonstrated a lack of difference in CPAP compliance between men and women,[29–32] increased compliance in women[33] as well as decreased compliance in women.[34–36] Regarding treatment efficacy, CPAP has been shown to improve insomnia symptoms in women more than men.[37] Men have demonstrated more profoundly increased health-related quality-of-life scores than women with CPAP treatment,[32] and CPAP treatment has been associated with lower mortality rates in male individuals with OSA compared to female individuals.[38] Finally, regarding CPAP settings, men may need higher levels of CPAP than women with the same OSA severity.[39,40]

Oral Appliance Therapy

Oral appliances enhance the upper airway structure and guard against airway collapse by adjusting the positioning of the jaw and tongue. Data suggest that individuals who are less obese,[41] have smaller neck circumferences,[42] lower baseline AHI,[43] and reduced upper airway collapsibility[44] may benefit more from oral appliances. Female sex has been reported as a predictor of success with oral appliance therapy (OAT)[45,46] which may be attributed to a reduced pharyngeal fat distribution and upper airway collapsibility[47] observed in female patients. Together, such data suggest that younger female patients with lower AHI may be the ideal candidates to trial OAT.

Hormone Replacement Therapy

Given the intersection of OSA with sex hormones and a higher prevalence of OSA in postmenopausal women, HRT has been studied as a possible treatment of OSA.

Bixler and colleagues found a near 4-fold increased risk of developing OSA in postmenopausal women without HRT as compared to premenopausal women and postmenopausal women receiving HRT.[16] Several researchers have demonstrated a reduction in mean AHI on estrogen therapy[48] or combined estrogen and progesterone therapy[49,50]; however, these studies were in a small sample of postmenopausal women. In a placebo-controlled double-blinded trial of postmenopausal women, the investigators found that initiation of medroxyprogesterone acetate in combination with discontinuation of nasal CPAP had increased nocturnal oxygen saturation and decreased arterial carbon dioxide; however, patients had an overall increase in AHI.[30] Other large cohort studies have shown no significant effect of HRT on OSA in postmenopausal women.[11] Ultimately, studies investigating the impact of HRT on OSA are sparse and limited by small sample sizes and varying HRT treatments; given the lack of definitive data and considerable side effects, HRT is not currently recommended as a treatment for OSA.[51]

Surgery

For adults with OSA who cannot tolerate CPAP, several surgical options exist that may significantly improve disease severity and/or improve CPAP tolerance. Typical surgical interventions for OSA include nasal surgery, palate surgery including uvulopalatopharyngoplasty, lingual tonsillectomy, midline glossectomy, transoral robotic surgery, genioglossus advancement, maxillomandibular advancement, hypoglossal nerve stimulation, and even tracheostomy. Unfortunately, most studies that have looked at the efficacy of surgical interventions for treatment of OSA have disproportionately included men[52] and the role of sex has not been well described. There are emerging data that suggest female patients may have increased success with upper airway stimulation (UAS) procedures as defined by a reduction in AHI and increase in device compliance.[53] Additionally, many surgical interventions rely on failed CPAP usage and severity of disease based on AHI for third party payment coverage. Recent data suggest that women may miss this cutoff given they present with lower AHI on average and, therefore, may handicap surgeons from offering the full array of procedures for OSA treatment.[54] Ultimately, the data on sex-specific surgical treatment are an area of future research.

In summary, OSA is more prevalent in men than women likely due to differences in craniofacial anatomy, fat distribution patterns, and hormonal factors. There are also sex-specific differences in OSA symptoms that can lead to underdiagnosis of OSA in women who are more likely to present with fatigue-related symptoms. OSA treatment options are similar for men and women, but some potential sex-specific differences in responsiveness to treatment have been noted including men responding better to weight loss and women responding better to OAT and possibly UAS (**Table 1**). More studies are needed to better assess sex-specific differences in responsiveness to various OSA treatments.

OBSTRUCTIVE SLEEP APNEA IN PREGNANCY

The overall prevalence of OSA during mid-to-late pregnancy is around 15%[55] which represents a 3 fold increase in the stated prevalence of OSA in women of reproductive age.[56] Several factors contribute to this finding including narrowed upper airway dimensions,[57] increased estrogen levels causing mucosal edema, nasal congestion and rhinitis of pregnancy, decreased functional capacity, increased oxygen consumption, and overall weight gain (**Fig. 1**). There are 2 phenotypes of OSA in pregnancy including women with preexisting OSA that become pregnant and women who

Table 1
Obstructive sleep apnea treatment differences between men and women

Treatment	Gender Differences
Weight loss	• May be more effective in *men* in reducing objective measures of sleep-disordered breathing • No defined difference regarding effectiveness of bariatric surgery
Oral appliance therapy	• *Women* may have increased success with OAT in reducing apnea–hypopnea index
Continuous positive airway pressure	• No defined difference on compliance • CPAP has been found to be associated with lower mortality rates in *men* • *Men* may need higher levels of CPAP after adjusting for OSA severity
Hormone replacement therapy	• No significant effect of HRT on OSA in postmenopausal women • Not currently recommended as a treatment for OSA
Surgery	• Most studies on sleep surgery have been performed in men • Emerging data suggest that *women* may have increase success with upper airway stimulation procedures

Abbreviations: CPAP, continuous positive airway pressure; HRT, hormone replacement therapy; OAT, oral appliance therapy; OSA, obstructive sleep apnea.

develop OSA during pregnancy. Studies suggest that the latter phenotype could potentially improve or fully resolve following childbirth, much like other systemic pregnancy-related conditions.[58] Both of these phenotypes progress throughout pregnancy with studies demonstrating the prevalence of OSA may double between early to late pregnancy.[59,60] Increased age and BMI have been found to be the most significant risk factors for more severe OSA in pregnant women.[59] The prevalence of OSA in

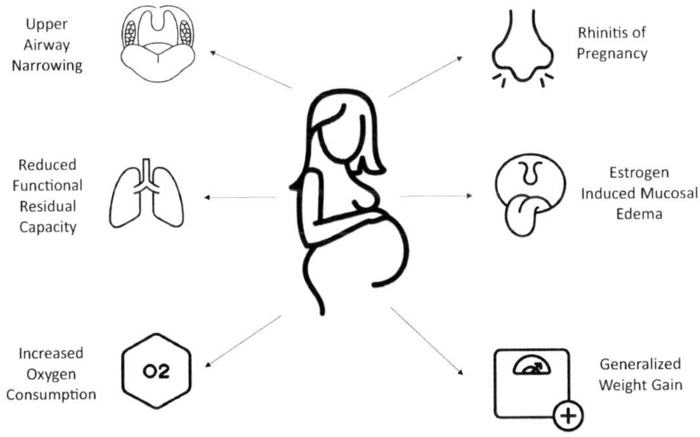

Fig. 1. Physiologic factors leading to increased prevalence of obstructive sleep apnea in pregnancy. Individual icons sourced from The Noun Project: Pregnant by Rifai; Tonsils by Amethyst Studio; Lung by Cuputo; O2 by Foodicons Collection; Flu by Vectors point; Tonsils by Sergey Demushkin point; Gain weight by DailyPM.

pregnancy will likely increase alongside rising rates of obesity and advanced maternal age.

Adverse Maternal and Fetal Outcomes

Compared to pregnant women without OSA, pregnant women with OSA have increased risk of pregnancy-specific complications including gestational hypertension, diabetes, increased hospital stays including increased odds of intensive care unit admission[61] and overall mortality.[62] In a large retrospective cohort study, the investigators found that pregnant women with OSA had a 5 fold increased risk of dying prior to discharge even after adjusting for serious cardiovascular, renal, and metabolic conditions that are known to affect mortality.[62] In addition to adverse maternal outcomes, OSA in pregnancy has been shown to put the fetus at risk as well. Pregnant women with OSA are at an increased risk of having infants with congenital anomalies[63] and low birth weight.[61] They also have higher rates of preterm[63] labor and cesarean sections.[64] Additional data suggest that maternal OSA may continue to impact the child later in life including increased hospitalizations in the first year of life, increasing special needs status and lower numeric test scores during school aged years.[65]

Unique Diagnostic Challenges

The well-validated OSA screening tools in pregnancy are sparse, and there is no consensus on the optimal time to initiate screening. In their review of screening questionnaires of OSA in pregnancy, Tantrakul and colleagues found that the Berlin questionnaire and Epworth Sleepiness Scale (ESS) were the most frequently used screening tools during pregnancy, with the Berlin questionnaire having poor-to-fair performance and the ESS having a very poor predictive value for diagnosing OSA.[66] Explanations for this include the comorbid sleep disturbances as well as the dynamic changes in symptomatology that occur throughout pregnancy. Ideally, after appropriate screening, women would get referred for a polysomnography (PSG) which is the gold standard for OSA diagnosis. Unfortunately, PSGs are expensive and often have relatively long wait times, making the diagnosis difficult to obtain during a pregnancy. Home sleep testing is emerging as a convenient, feasible method for diagnosing OSA in high-risk populations. Emerging data have shown the efficacy of portable devices as compared to PSG in diagnosing OSA in pregnant women. Specifically, the Apnea Risk Evaluation System,[67] Watch-PAT-200 wrist-worn screening tool,[68] and Nox-T3 portable monitor[69] demonstrated strong sensitivity and specificity in detecting OSA in pregnant women.

TREATMENT OPTIONS

Continuous Positive Airway Pressure in Pregnancy

In line with nonpregnant women, CPAP is the first-line treatment for OSA in pregnancy. CPAP has been shown to be effective in improving symptoms of sleep-disordered breathing in pregnancy including sleepiness, fatigue and snoring[70] as well as blood pressure,[66] heart rate, and cardiac stroke volume in women with preeclampsia.[71] In a systematic review of CPAP in pregnancy, researchers concluded that CPAP initiation is safe and relatively well tolerated in pregnancy. They also noted that CPAP may reduce blood pressure, preeclampsia, preterm birth, and increase neonatal birth weight; however, the overall evidence was of low quality and further prospective randomized trials are needed on this topic.[72] Of note, auto-CPAP has specific advantages in treating women with OSA given the faster initiation of therapy and ability to autotitrate CPAP to accommodate the weight gain and upper airway alterations that occur throughout pregnancy.[70]

Alternative Treatment Options

Conservative treatment options include control of pregnancy-related weight gain, sleeping in the lateral position, and head of bed elevation during sleep.[73] In contrast to OSA management in the nonpregnant population, excessive weight loss is not generally recommended given the potential harm to the fetus. OAT may be considered in pregnancy when CPAP is not tolerated or is contraindicated. However, OAT feasibility during pregnancy is diminished due to the limited likelihood of timely intervention given these devices can take up to several months to create with multiple fitting appointments needed.[74] Elective surgical interventions are contraindicated due to the maternal and fetal risk of general anesthesia.

The Otolaryngologist's Role in Treating Obstructive Sleep Apnea in Pregnancy

Generally, otolaryngologists are not involved in the screening and management of OSA in pregnancy; however, they can still play an important role, such as in the management of rhinitis.

Rhinitis of Pregnancy

Rhinitis of pregnancy is defined as nasal obstruction in the last 6 or more weeks of gestation without a known allergic cause with complete resolution after delivery.[75] It has been shown to have an estimated prevalence ranging from 9%[76] to 40%.[77] Both allergic and nonallergic rhinitis have been identified as risk factors for OSA,[78] and management of rhinitis may benefit patients by improving sleep quality and CPAP tolerance.[79] Treatment of pregnancy rhinitis can include increased physical exercise, head and bed elevation, nasal dilators, and saline sprays for temporary relieve. Saline nasal sprays are safe, have been shown to reduce rhinitis symptoms in pregnancy, and should be considered a first-line treatment.[80] Intranasal corticosteroids, with the exception of triamcinolone, are generally considered safe in pregnancy. The most widely studied intranasal steroid in pregnancy is budesonide, specifically 50 μg applied to each nostril up to twice per day.[81] However, intranasal corticosteroids have not been found to be an effective treatment for rhinitis in pregnancy.[82] Topical decongestants are considered class C drugs, indicating that there were some side effects for the fetus in animal experiments, but the benefit may justify the potential risk during pregnancy. Studies have shown an increased risk of developing pyloric stenosis in first trimester and renal collecting system anomalies in the second trimester with usage of intranasal decongestants; however, the authors admit their findings may have been altered by recall bias and the absolute risk remains small.[83] Anecdotal evidence supports the use of ipratropium bromide (0.03%) nasal spray for pregnancy rhinitis associated with significant rhinorrhea,[84] and it is considered safe in pregnancy.[75]

Allergic Rhinitis in Pregnancy

Pregnancy may also exacerbate preexisting allergic rhinitis. In addition to allergen avoidance, intranasal cromolyn is generally recommended as the first-line treatment for pregnant patients with allergic rhinitis given its excellent safety profile likely related to low circulating plasma levels.[85] Second-generation antihistamines are also generally considered safe and effective treatments.[86,87] Azelastine is a category C drug with no adequate and well-controlled studies in human participants. Finally, allergen immunotherapy should not be newly started in pregnant women, though it is generally recommended to be continued if it has already been initiated and the patient is showing benefit.[88]

In-office inferior turbinate reduction has been described as a treatment for rhinitis of pregnancy[75] and successfully used by the authors for symptomatic treatment of refractory nasal congestion. Given the low risk and lack of systemic effects of this procedure, it should be considered more commonly when symptoms are refractory to medical therapy. Of note, inferior turbinate radiofrequency ablation has been shown to improve CPAP compliance[89] as nasal obstruction is one of the most commonly stated reasons for CPAP intolerance.

Postpartum Management

OSA precipitated by pregnancy usually improves after delivery, but women diagnosed with OSA during pregnancy should be followed postpartum to determine whether OSA has resolved or requires further treatment. Little is known about how frequently OSA during pregnancy persists in the postpartum period or how gestational OSA impacts cardiovascular risks later in life.[90]

Withdrawal of CPAP can be attempted in mild–moderate pregnancy-associated OSA if symptoms have improved postpartum. Researchers recommend continuing CPAP for severe pregnancy-associated sleep apnea until weight returns to 10% to 15% of baseline and repeat PSG should be obtained at that time. Women with gestational OSA should be monitored closely for the development of OSA in subsequent pregnancies.[91] Women with preexisting OSA or gestational OSA that does not resolve after delivery and who desire additional children may represent an important population. In this scenario, surgical intervention can be timed outside of pregnancy and may prevent future adverse maternal and fetal outcomes.

In conclusion, the complex interaction between OSA and pregnancy presents a challenge in health care. The prevalence of OSA during pregnancy is increased primarily due to various physiologic changes associated with gestation. This condition not only places pregnant women at risk of complications but also affects fetal health with potential long-term consequences for the child. The diagnostic landscape for OSA in pregnancy is challenging, with the need for improved screening tools and timely diagnostic methods. CPAP remains a cornerstone treatment for OSA in pregnancy, with evidence suggesting its benefits for both maternal and fetal well-being. Moving forward, it is crucial to address OSA in pregnant women comprehensively, considering the unique aspects of this population and to conduct further research to refine diagnostic and therapeutic strategies.

CLINICS CARE POINTS

- Obstructive sleep apnea (OSA) is more prevalent in men than women. Women may have atypical presentations of OSA, including nonspecific symptoms like fatigue and insomnia, which can lead to underdiagnosis.
- After menopause, there is a notable increase in OSA prevalence in women. Menopause-related hormonal changes, including decreased estrogen and progesterone levels, can contribute to the development of OSA. Hormone replacement therapy has been explored as a treatment option, but its effectiveness remains inconclusive.
- Sex-specific treatment responses in OSA exist; however, further research is needed on this topic.
- The rates of OSA are higher in pregnant patients than in the nonpregnant population due to hormonal and anatomic changes during pregnancy.

- Home sleep apnea testing may be a reasonable diagnostic alterative to PSG in pregnant patients with suspected OSA to facilitate expedited and streamlined diagnosis and management.
- While otolaryngologists may not typically be involved in OSA screening and management during pregnancy, they can have a meaningful impact by addressing rhinitis-related symptoms, which can indirectly improve sleep quality and continuous positive airway pressure tolerance, as well as evaluating for surgical candidacy prior to future pregnancies.

DISCLOSURE

The authors have no relevant disclosures.

REFERENCES

1. Senaratna CV, Perret JL, Lodge CJ, et al. Prevalence of obstructive sleep apnea in the general population: A systematic review. Sleep Med Rev 2017;34. https://doi.org/10.1016/j.smrv.2016.07.002.
2. Franklin KA, Lindberg E. Obstructive sleep apnea is a common disorder in the population-A review on the epidemiology of sleep apnea. J Thorac Dis 2015; 7(8). https://doi.org/10.3978/j.issn.2072-1439.2015.06.11.
3. Shepertycky MR, Banno K, Kryger MH. Differences between men and women in the clinical presentation of patients diagnosed with obstructive sleep apnea syndrome. Sleep 2005;28(3). https://doi.org/10.1016/s8756-3452(08)70176-2.
4. Malhotra A, Huang Y, Fogel RB, et al. The male predisposition to pharyngeal collapse: Importance of airway length. Am J Respir Crit Care Med 2002; 166(10). https://doi.org/10.1164/rccm.2112072.
5. Segal Y, Malhotra A, Pillar G. Upper airway length may be associated with the severity of obstructive sleep apnea syndrome. Sleep Breath 2008;12(4). https://doi.org/10.1007/s11325-008-0191-9.
6. Pillar G, Lavie P. Psychiatric symptoms in sleep apnea syndrome: Effects of gender and respiratory disturbance index. Chest 1998;114(3). https://doi.org/10.1378/chest.114.3.697.
7. Wahner-Roedler DL, Olson EJ, Narayanan S, et al. Gender-specific differences in a patient population with obstructive sleep apnea-hypopnea syndrome. Gend Med 2007;4(4). https://doi.org/10.1016/S1550-8579(07)80062-3.
8. Cairns A, Poulos G, Bogan R. Sex differences in sleep apnea predictors and outcomes from home sleep apnea testing. Nat Sci Sleep 2016;8. https://doi.org/10.2147/NSS.S101186.
9. Kapsimalis F, Kryger MH. Gender and obstructive sleep apnea syndrome, part 1: Clinical features. Sleep 2002;25(4). https://doi.org/10.1093/sleep/25.4.409.
10. Valipour A, Lothaller H, Rauscher H, et al. Gender-related differences in symptoms of patients with suspected breathing disorders in sleep: A clinical population study using the Sleep Disorders Questionnaire. Sleep 2007;30(3). https://doi.org/10.1093/sleep/30.3.312.
11. Young T, Hutton R, Finn L, et al. The gender bias in sleep apnea diagnosis: Are women missed because they have different symptoms? Arch Intern Med 1996; 156(21). https://doi.org/10.1001/archinte.156.21.2445.
12. Quintana-Gallego E, Carmona-Bernal C, Capote F, et al. Gender differences in obstructive sleep apnea syndrome: A clinical study of 1166 patients. Respir Med 2004;98(10). https://doi.org/10.1016/j.rmed.2004.03.002.

13. Redline S, Kump K, Tishler PV, et al. Gender differences in sleep disordered breathing in a community-based sample. Am J Respir Crit Care Med 1994; 149(3 I). https://doi.org/10.1164/ajrccm.149.3.8118642.
14. Krishnan V, Collop NA. Gender differences in sleep disorders. Curr Opin Pulm Med 2006;12(6):383–9.
15. Block AJ, Wynne JW, Boysen PG. Sleep-disordered breathing and nocturnal oxygen desaturation in postmenopausal women. Am J Med 1980;69(1). https://doi.org/10.1016/0002-9343(80)90502-1.
16. Bixler EO, Vgontzas AN, Lin HM, et al. Prevalence of sleep-disordered breathing in women: Effects of gender. Am J Respir Crit Care Med 2001;163(3 I). https://doi.org/10.1164/ajrccm.163.3.9911064.
17. Netzer NC, Eliasson AH, Strohl KP. Women with sleep apnea have lower levels of sex hormones. Sleep Breath 2003;7(1). https://doi.org/10.1007/s11325-003-0025-8.
18. Popovic RM, White DP. Upper airway muscle activity in normal women: Influence of hormonal status. J Appl Physiol 1998;84(3). https://doi.org/10.1152/jappl.1998.84.3.1055.
19. Dancey DR, Hanly PJ, Soong C, et al. Impact of menopause on the prevalence and severity of sleep apnea. Chest 2001;120(1). https://doi.org/10.1378/chest.120.1.151.
20. Thurnheer R, Wraith PK, Douglas NJ. Influence of age and gender on upper airway resistance in NREM and REM sleep. J Appl Physiol 2001;90(3). https://doi.org/10.1152/jappl.2001.90.3.981.
21. Chooi YC, Ding C, Magkos F. The epidemiology of obesity. Metabolism 2019;92. https://doi.org/10.1016/j.metabol.2018.09.005.
22. Huang KT, Chin CH, Tseng CC, et al. The Influence of Obesity on Different Genders in Patients with Obstructive Sleep Apnea. Sci World J 2014;2014. https://doi.org/10.1155/2014/487215.
23. Valadares RJB, Sousa KG, Espindola MN, et al. Gender Differences in Comorbidities and Sleep Patterns of Obese Patients with Obstructive Sleep Apnea. World J Neurosci 2015;05(01). https://doi.org/10.4236/wjns.2015.51006.
24. Resta O, Carpagnano GE, Lacedonia D, et al. Gender difference in sleep profile of severely obese patients with obstructive sleep apnea (OSA). Respir Med 2005; 99(1). https://doi.org/10.1016/j.rmed.2004.05.014.
25. Newman AB, Nieto FJ, Guidry U, et al. Relation of sleep-disordered breathing to cardiovascular disease risk factors: The Sleep Heart Health Study. Am J Epidemiol 2001;154(1). https://doi.org/10.1093/aje/154.1.50.
26. Newman AB, Foster G, Givelber R, et al. Progression and regression of sleep-disordered breathing with changes in weight: The Sleep Heart Health Study. Arch Intern Med 2005;165(20). https://doi.org/10.1001/archinte.165.20.2408.
27. Sarkhosh K, Switzer NJ, El-Hadi M, et al. The impact of bariatric surgery on obstructive sleep apnea: A systematic review. Obes Surg 2013;23(3). https://doi.org/10.1007/s11695-012-0862-2.
28. Kennedy-Dalby A, Adam S, Ammori BJ, et al. Weight loss and metabolic outcomes of bariatric surgery in men versus women - A matched comparative observational cohort study. Eur J Intern Med 2014;25(10). https://doi.org/10.1016/j.ejim.2014.10.020.
29. Budhiraja R, Parthasarathy S, Drake CL, et al. Early CPAP use identifies subsequent adherence to CPAP therapy. Sleep 2007;30(3). https://doi.org/10.1016/s8756-3452(08)70706-0.

30. Anttalainen U, Saaresranta T, Kalleinen N, et al. CPAP adherence and partial upper airway obstruction during sleep. Sleep Breath 2007;11(3). https://doi.org/10.1007/s11325-007-0102-5.
31. Ye L, Pien GW, Weaver TE. Gender differences in the clinical manifestation of obstructive sleep apnea. Sleep Med 2009;10(10). https://doi.org/10.1016/j.sleep.2009.02.006.
32. Lo Bue A, Salvaggio A, Iacono Isidoro S, et al. OSA and CPAP therapy: effect of gender, somnolence, and treatment adherence on health-related quality of life. Sleep Breath 2020;24(2). https://doi.org/10.1007/s11325-019-01895-3.
33. Sin DD, Mayers I, Man GCW, et al. Long-term compliance rates to continuous positive airway pressure in obstructive sleep apnea a population-based study. Chest 2002;121(2). https://doi.org/10.1378/chest.121.2.430.
34. Pelletier-Fleury N, Rakotonanahary D, Fleury B. The age and other factors in the evaluation of compliance with nasal continuous positive airway pressure for obstructive sleep apnea syndrome. A Cox's proportional hazard analysis. Sleep Med 2001;2(3). https://doi.org/10.1016/S1389-9457(00)00063-0.
35. Woehrle H, Graml A, Weinreich G. Age- and gender-dependent adherence with continuous positive airway pressure therapy. Sleep Med 2011;12(10). https://doi.org/10.1016/j.sleep.2011.05.008.
36. Huang YC, Lan CC, Wu YK, et al. Age- and gender-related differences of CPAP acceptance for obstructive sleep apnea syndrome in Taiwan. Sleep Biol Rhythms 2018;16(1). https://doi.org/10.1007/s41105-017-0132-8.
37. Loução-De-Amorim I, Bentes C, Peralta AR. Men and women with chronic insomnia disorder and OSAS: Different responses to CPAP. Sleep Science 2019;12. https://doi.org/10.5935/1984-0063.20190085.
38. Jennum P, Tønnesen P, Ibsen R, et al. All-cause mortality from obstructive sleep apnea in male and female patients with and without continuous positive airway pressure treatment: a registry study with 10 years of follow-up. Nat Sci Sleep 2015;7:43–50.
39. Jayaraman G, Majid H, Surani S, et al. Influence of gender on continuous positive airway pressure requirements in patients with obstructive sleep apnea syndrome. Sleep Breath 2011;15(4). https://doi.org/10.1007/s11325-010-0436-2.
40. Yukawa K, Inoue Y, Yagyu H, et al. Gender differences in the clinical characteristics among japanese patients with obstructive sleep apnea syndrome. Chest 2009;135(2). https://doi.org/10.1378/chest.08-1414.
41. Otsuka R, De Almeida FR, Lowe AA, et al. A comparison of responders and nonresponders to oral appliance therapy for the treatment of obstructive sleep apnea. Am J Orthod Dentofacial Orthop 2006;129(2). https://doi.org/10.1016/j.ajodo.2004.06.035.
42. Barnes M, McEvoy RD, Banks S, et al. Efficacy of positive airway pressure and oral appliance in mild to moderate obstructive sleep apnea. Am J Respir Crit Care Med 2004;170(6). https://doi.org/10.1164/rccm.200311-1571OC.
43. Mehta A, Qian J, Petocz P, et al. A randomized, controlled study of a mandibular advancement splint for obstructive sleep apnea. Am J Respir Crit Care Med 2001;163(6). https://doi.org/10.1164/ajrccm.163.6.2004213.
44. Edwards BA, Andara C, Landry S, et al. Upper-airway collapsibility and loop gain predict the response to oral appliance therapy in patients with obstructive sleep apnea. Am J Respir Crit Care Med 2016;194(11). https://doi.org/10.1164/rccm.201601-0099OC.
45. Marklund M, Stenlund H, Franklin KA. Mandibular advancement devices in 630 men and women with obstructive sleep apnea and snoring: Tolerability and

predictors of treatment success. Chest 2004;125(4). https://doi.org/10.1378/chest.125.4.1270.

46. Vecchierini MF, Attali V, Collet JM, et al. Sex differences in mandibular repositioning device therapy effectiveness in patients with obstructive sleep apnea syndrome. Sleep Breath 2019;23(3). https://doi.org/10.1007/s11325-018-1766-8.
47. Mohsenin V. Effects of gender on upper airway collapsibility and severity of obstructive sleep apnea. Sleep Med 2003;4(6). https://doi.org/10.1016/S1389-9457(03)00168-0.
48. Manber R, Kuo TF, Cataldo N, et al. The effects of hormone replacement therapy on sleep-disordered breathing in postmenopausal women: A pilot study. Sleep 2003;26(2). https://doi.org/10.1093/sleep/26.2.163.
49. Pickett CK, Regensteiner JG, Woodard WD, et al. Progestin and estrogen reduce sleep-disordered breathing in postmenopausal women. J Appl Physiol 1989;66(4). https://doi.org/10.1152/jappl.1989.66.4.1656.
50. Wesström J, Uufberg J, Nilsson S. Sleep apnea and hormone replacement therapy: A pilot study and a literature review. Acta Obstet Gynecol Scand 2005;84(1). https://doi.org/10.1111/j.0001-6349.2005.00575.x.
51. Lindberg E, Bonsignore MR, Polo-Kantola P. Role of menopause and hormone replacement therapy in sleep-disordered breathing. Sleep Med Rev 2020;49. https://doi.org/10.1016/j.smrv.2019.101225.
52. Debbaneh P, Ramirez K, Block-Wheeler N, et al. Representation of Race and Sex in Sleep Surgery Studies. Otolaryngol Head Neck Surg 2022;166(6). https://doi.org/10.1177/01945998221088759.
53. Thaler E, Schwab R, Maurer J, et al. Results of the ADHERE upper airway stimulation registry and predictors of therapy efficacy. Laryngoscope 2020;130(5). https://doi.org/10.1002/lary.28286.
54. Chang CP, Dierks E, Cheng A, et al. Does the Lack of Gender-Specific Apnea-Hypopnea Index Cutoff for Obstructive Sleep Apnea Impact Surgical Selection? J Oral Maxillofac Surg 2021;79(3). https://doi.org/10.1016/j.joms.2020.11.001.
55. Liu L, Su G, Wang S, et al. The prevalence of obstructive sleep apnea and its association with pregnancy-related health outcomes: a systematic review and meta-analysis. Sleep Breath 2019;23(2). https://doi.org/10.1007/s11325-018-1714-7.
56. Young T, Palta M, Dempsey J, et al. The Occurrence of Sleep-Disordered Breathing among Middle-Aged Adults. N Engl J Med 1993;328(17). https://doi.org/10.1056/nejm199304293281704.
57. Izci B, Vennelle M, Liston WA, et al. Sleep-disordered breathing and upper airway size in pregnancy and post-partum. Eur Respir J 2006;27(2). https://doi.org/10.1183/09031936.06.00148204.
58. Reid J, Glew RA, Skomro R, et al. Sleep disordered breathing and gestational hypertension: Postpartum follow-up study. Sleep 2013;36(5). https://doi.org/10.5665/sleep.2634.
59. Pien GW, Pack AI, Jackson N, et al. Risk factors for sleep-disordered breathing in pregnancy. Thorax 2014;69(4). https://doi.org/10.1136/thoraxjnl-2012-202718.
60. Facco FL, Parker CB, Reddy UM, et al. Association between Sleep-Disordered Breathing and Hypertensive Disorders of Pregnancy and Gestational Diabetes Mellitus. Obstet Gynecol 2017;129. https://doi.org/10.1097/AOG.0000000000001805.
61. Bourjeily G, Danilack VA, Bublitz MH, et al. Obstructive sleep apnea in pregnancy is associated with adverse maternal outcomes: a national cohort. Sleep Med 2017;38. https://doi.org/10.1016/j.sleep.2017.06.035.

62. Louis JM, Mogos MF, Salemi JL, et al. Obstructive sleep apnea and severe maternal-infant morbidity/mortality in the United states, 1998-2009. Sleep 2014; 37(5). https://doi.org/10.5665/sleep.3644.
63. Bourjeily G, Danilack VA, Bublitz MH, et al. Maternal obstructive sleep apnea and neonatal birth outcomes in a population based sample. Sleep Med 2020;66. https://doi.org/10.1016/j.sleep.2019.01.019.
64. Chen YH, Kang JH, Lin CC, et al. Obstructive sleep apnea and the risk of adverse pregnancy outcomes. Am J Obstet Gynecol 2012;206(2). https://doi.org/10.1016/j.ajog.2011.09.006.
65. Bin YS, Cistulli PA, Roberts CL, et al. Childhood health and educational outcomes associated with maternal sleep apnea: A population record-linkage study. Sleep 2017;40(11). https://doi.org/10.1093/sleep/zsx158.
66. Tantrakul V, Numthavaj P, Guilleminault C, et al. Performance of screening questionnaires for obstructive sleep apnea during pregnancy: A systematic review and meta-analysis. Sleep Med Rev 2017;36. https://doi.org/10.1016/j.smrv.2016.11.003.
67. Sharkey KM, Waters K, Millman RP, et al. Validation of the Apnea Risk Evaluation System (ARES) device against laboratory polysomnography in pregnant women at risk for obstructive sleep apnea syndrome. J Clin Sleep Med 2014;10(5). https://doi.org/10.5664/jcsm.3694.
68. O'Brien LM, Bullough AS, Shelgikar AV, et al. Validation of watch-PAT-200 against polysomnography during pregnancy. J Clin Sleep Med 2012;8(3). https://doi.org/10.5664/jcsm.1916.
69. Wang J, Zhang C, Xu L, et al. Home monitoring for clinically suspected obstructive sleep apnea in pregnancy. J Clin Sleep Med 2023;19(11):1951–60.
70. Guilleminault C, Kreutzer M, Chang JL. Pregnancy, sleep disordered breathing and treatment with nasal continuous positive airway pressure. Sleep Med 2004; 5(1). https://doi.org/10.1016/j.sleep.2003.07.001.
71. Blyton DM, Sullivan CE, Edwards N. Reduced nocturnal cardiac output associated with preeclampsia is minimized with the use of nocturnal nasal CPAP. Sleep 2004;27(1). https://doi.org/10.1093/sleep/27.1.79.
72. Nugent R, Wee A, Kearney L, et al. The effectiveness of continuous positive airway pressure for treating obstructive sleep apnoea in pregnancy: A systematic review. Aust N Z J Obstet Gynaecol 2023;63(3). https://doi.org/10.1111/ajo.13654.
73. Kapsimalis F, Kryger M. Obstructive Sleep Apnea in Pregnancy. Sleep Med Clin 2007;2(4). https://doi.org/10.1016/j.jsmc.2007.07.002.
74. Erdem D, Şevik Eliçora S, Passali GC. Snoring and Sleep Apnea During Pregnancy and Postpartum Period. In: Cingi C, Özel HE, Bayar Muluk N, editors ENT, editors. Diseases: Diagnosis and Treatment during Pregnancy and Lactation. Cham.: Springer; 2022. https://doi.org/10.1007/978-3-031-05303-0_17.
75. Orban N, Maughan E, Bleach N. Pregnancy-induced rhinitis. Rhinology 2013; 51(2). https://doi.org/10.4193/Rhino12.045.
76. Shushan S, Sadan O, Lurie S, et al. Pregnancy-associated rhinitis. Am J Perinatol 2006;23(7). https://doi.org/10.1055/s-2006-951302.
77. Ulkumen B, Artunc Ulkumen B, Pala HG, et al. Pregnancy rhinitis in Turkish women: Do gestational week, BMI and parity affect nasal congestion? Pak J Med Sci 2016;32(4). https://doi.org/10.12669/pjms.324.10164.

78. Kalpaklioğlu AF, Kavut AB, Ekici M. Allergic and nonallergic rhinitis: The threat for obstructive sleep apnea. Ann Allergy Asthma Immunol 2009;103(1). https://doi.org/10.1016/S1081-1206(10)60138-X.
79. Fueyo GO. Chronic Rhinitis Treatment: Effects on Obstructive Sleep Apnea. Curr Treat Options Allergy 2022;9(3). https://doi.org/10.1007/s40521-022-00307-4.
80. Garavello W, Somigliana E, Acaia B, et al. Nasal lavage in pregnant women with seasonal allergic rhinitis: A randomized study. Int Arch Allergy Immunol 2010; 151(2). https://doi.org/10.1159/000236003.
81. Norjavaara E, De Verdier MG. Normal pregnancy outcomes in a population-based study including 2968 pregnant women exposed to budesonide. J Allergy Clin Immunol 2003;111(4). https://doi.org/10.1067/mai.2003.1340.
82. Ellegård EK, Hellgren M, Karlsson NG. Fluticasone propionate aqueous nasal spray in pregnancy rhinitis. Clin Otolaryngol Allied Sci 2001;26(5). https://doi.org/10.1046/j.1365-2273.2001.00491.x.
83. Yau WP, Mitchell AA, Lin KJ, et al. Use of decongestants during pregnancy and the risk of birth defects. Am J Epidemiol 2013;178(2). https://doi.org/10.1093/aje/kws427.
84. Namazy JA, Schatz M. Diagnosing Rhinitis during Pregnancy. Curr Allergy Asthma Rep 2014;14(9). https://doi.org/10.1007/s11882-014-0458-0.
85. Sato K. Treatment of allergic rhinitis during pregnancy. Clin Exp Allergy Rev 2012; 12(1). https://doi.org/10.1111/j.1472-9733.2011.01160.x.
86. Källén B. Use of antihistamine drugs in early pregnancy and delivery outcome. J Matern Fetal Neonatal Med 2002;11(3). https://doi.org/10.1080/jmf.11.3.146.152.
87. Diav-Citrin O, Shechtman S, Aharonovich A, et al. Pregnancy outcome after gestational exposure to loratadine or antihistamines: A prospective controlled cohort study. J Allergy Clin Immunol 2003;111(6). https://doi.org/10.1067/mai.2003.1499.
88. Khan NU, Begum KS. Allergic Rhinitis during Pregnancy -an Update of Management. Med Today 2017;28(2). https://doi.org/10.3329/medtoday.v28i2.32933.
89. Elwany S, Bahgat AY, Ibrahim M, et al. Surgical correction of nasal obstruction in obstructive sleep apnea improves CPAP outcomes and compliance. Ir J Med Sci 2022;191(6). https://doi.org/10.1007/s11845-021-02896-6.
90. Chang JL, Goldberg AN, Alt JA, et al. International consensus statement on obstructive sleep apnea. Int Forum Allergy Rhinol 2023. https://doi.org/10.1002/alr.23079.
91. Venkata C, Venkateshiah SB. Sleep-disordered breathing during pregnancy. J Am Board Fam Med 2009;22(2):158–68.

Positional Treatment of Obstructive Sleep Apnea

Madeline Jacqueline Louise Ravesloot, MD, PhD, MSc

KEYWORDS

- Obstructive sleep apnea • Positional sleep apnea • Positional therapy • Compliance
- Treatment effectiveness • New-generation positional therapy • Sleep position
- Disease severity

KEY POINTS

- Positional sleep apnea (POSA) is a subtype of obstructive sleep apnea where the severity of the condition is highly dependent on the patient's sleeping position.
- Compliance with positional therapy (PT) is essential for the effective management of POSA, as it significantly influences treatment success and disease alleviation.
- New-generation PT devices exhibit higher compliance rates and greater disease alleviation compared to traditional methods like the tennis ball technique.
- Avoiding the supine sleep position is a valuable therapeutic strategy for POSA, underlining the need for a personalized approach that considers the patient's unique needs.

INTRODUCTION

In recent years, our understanding of obstructive sleep apnea (OSA) has evolved, revealing a multifactorial nature characterized by various physiologic mechanisms (endotypes) and clinical presentations (phenotypes). These insights have led to a more refined classification of OSA and a deeper comprehension of its pathogenesis. Consequently, this has ushered in new approaches in both clinical decision-making and research, ultimately shifting the landscape of OSA treatment from a "one-size-fits-all" approach to personalized therapeutic interventions that target specific pathophysiological mechanisms.[1,2]

Among the various endotypes, a significant focus has been on the nonanatomical contributors, which interact with anatomic factors and the collapsibility of the upper airway (UA). These contributors include a low respiratory arousal threshold, where patients awaken prematurely in response to a reduction in UA lumen, a high loop gain associated with an oversensitive ventilatory control system, and inadequate

Funding: No funding.
Department of Otorhinolaryngology–Head and Neck Surgery, OLVG, Jan Tooropstraat 164, Amsterdam 1061AE, the Netherlands
E-mail address: m.j.l.ravesloot@olvg.nl

Otolaryngol Clin N Am 57 (2024) 481–490
https://doi.org/10.1016/j.otc.2024.01.002
oto.theclinics.com

responsiveness of the UA dilator muscles during sleep and UA collapse.[3] Eckert and colleagues[4] have elucidated these endotypic traits, emphasizing their potential clinical applications. On a different note, an important distinction arises between patients who exhibit position-dependent OSA (POSA) and those who do not. The concept of positional therapy (PT) hinges on this difference, with profound implications for clinical practice.[3–5]

DEFINITIONS

In positional patients (PPs), the frequency and duration of apneas are notably influenced by the patient's sleeping position, particularly in the supine position. Remarkably, positional OSA accounts for a significant portion of OSA patients, ranging from 56% to 75%, and is especially prevalent in individuals with mild to moderate disease (70%–80%).[6–10] On the other hand, non–positional patients (NPPs) experience breathing abnormalities consistently in both supine and nonsupine positions.[11] While changing sleep positions may not dramatically alter the severity of the disease in NPPs, it is important to note that even in these cases, avoiding the supine position can lead to a notable improvement. The supine position tends to worsen the severity of apneas and hypopneas in almost all OSA patients.[12]

Various criteria have been introduced to define PPs with POSA, with Cartwright's criteria being the most commonly used, requiring a 50% or more difference in the apnea index between supine and nonsupine positions.[13] Over time, modified versions of Cartwright's criteria have been developed, incorporating additional parameters such as the overall Apnea-Hypopnea Index (AHI), AHI in supine and nonsupine positions, and the time spent in different sleeping positions.[9,11,14–18] PPs can be further categorized into 2 subgroups: supine-predominant (spOSA) and supine-isolated (siOSA).[10] In spOSA, respiratory disturbances are primarily observed in the supine position, persisting in nonsupine positions. In contrast, siOSA patients exhibit normalized respiratory patterns when in nonsupine positions, with an AHI of less than 5 per hour (**Fig. 1**).

IMPACT OF SLEEP POSITION ON DISEASE SEVERITY

For patients with POSA, the influence of sleeping position on disease severity is substantial. Avoiding the supine position can completely eliminate the disease in patients with siOSA, while those with spOSA experience a significant improvement, though not a complete resolution of their condition.

Interestingly, in 26% to 38% of OSA patients and 36% to 54% of PPs, respiratory disturbances normalize when in nonsupine positions.[6,9,19] A study in South Korea revealed that a majority of patients meeting the criteria for POSA had spOSA, while a smaller percentage of patients were siOSA.[20] siOSA patients experienced fewer arousal events but poorer sleep quality and a higher prevalence of depression.[19] Notably, the introduction of the 2012 American Academy of Sleep Medicine–recommended hypopnea criteria led to an increase in the prevalence of OSA and a greater identification of siOSA patients who could benefit from PT.[21]

Additionally, research suggests that head position and neck angle, in addition to trunk position, can play a significant role in reducing UA collapsibility in some patients.[4,22,23] Furthermore, while less commonly acknowledged, position-dependency has been observed in central sleep apnea.[24–29]

It is worth noting that PPs tend to be younger and have a lower body mass index in comparison to NPPs.[6–8,10,30] However, a recent cross-sectional study reported a

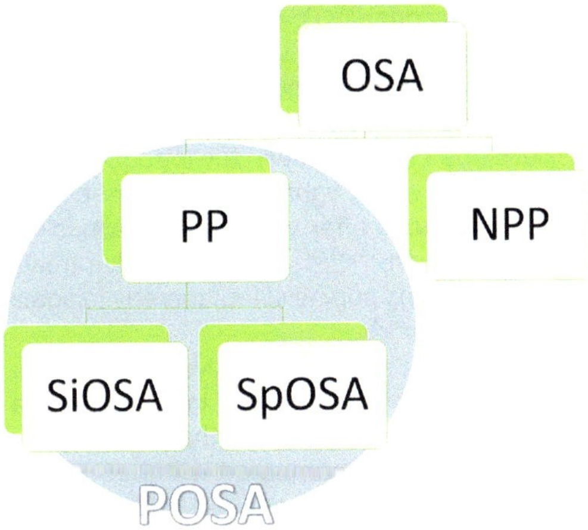

Fig. 1. Schematic overview definitions. (1) Patients with obstructive sleep apnea (OSA) can be divided into 2 groups: (a) In positional patients (PPs), desaturations, cyclic variations in heart rate, loud snoring, and apneas/hypopneas appear almost exclusively in the supine position. (b) In non-positional patients (NPPs), desaturations, cyclic variations in heart rate, loud snoring, and apneas/hypopneas appear independent of the body position. (2) PPs can be further be classified as (a) supine-predominant OSA (spOSA): In spOSA, respiratory disturbances are mainly in the supine position. These patients have persistent respiratory disturbances in nonsupine position. (b) Supine-isolated OSA (siOSA). In siOSA, respiratory disturbances normalize in the nonsupine position. (3) OSA patients who have an increase in breathing abnormalities while sleeping in the supine versus the lateral position are considered positional patients (PPs) and suffer from positional OSA (POSA). (*From* Ravesloot M, Vonk P, Maurer J, Oksenberg A, De Vries N. Standardized framework to report on the role of sleeping position in sleep apnea patients. Sleep and Breathing. 2021; 25:1717-1728.)

higher prevalence of severe POSA in patients aged greater than 65 years.[31] The prevalence of POSA has been noted to be higher in Asian populations.[20,32–34]

The distinction between PPs and NPPs carries essential therapeutic implications, and their identification is relatively straightforward, requiring a polysomnographic (PSG) or polygraphic study with continuous and accurate recording of sleeping position changes.

TREATMENT OF POSITIONAL OBSTRUCTIVE SLEEP APNEA

In PPs, avoiding the supine position is obviously a valuable therapeutic option in the management of this condition. Various techniques are described to prevent patients from assuming the supine position, such as an upright sleep posture, positional alarms, verbal instructions, and PT, the latter being the most effective and common.[10,35,36] In 1984, the *Chest* published a letter written by a patient's wife.[37] She had cured her husband's sleep apnea snoring problem by "having sewn a pocket into the back of a T-shirt and having inserted a hollow, lightweight plastic ball to prevent her husband sleeping on his back." During the American War of Independence (1775–1783) and later during World War I (1914–1918), soldiers were advised to wear their rucksacks (filled with a bulky mass) while sleeping in order to avoid sleeping on their backs and reduce snoring so as to avoid making their position known to the enemy.[38] PT, in whichever form, has been found to have a significant influence on snoring and OSA severity. These are early examples of the PT technique, commonly known as the tennis ball technique (TBT): a bulky object typically attached at the level of the upper back, such as a tennis ball, vests, "shark fins," and special pillows. The discomfort caused by the presence of the bulky mass discourages the patient from sleeping in the supine position but is also linked to poor (long-term) compliance.[38]

Therefore, recent developments have seen the introduction of a more modern new-generation PT, which involves small, lightweight, battery-powered devices affixed to the neck or chest. These devices offer vibrotactile feedback to patients when they adopt a supine sleeping position.[14,35,38,39] Both of these treatment modalities have demonstrated efficacy in reducing supine sleep, thereby mitigating obstructive events associated with this position.[35,36,38]

A recent systematic review and meta-analysis was published of randomized controlled trials (RCTs) and cohort studies that investigated the effect of vibrotactile PT in POSA patients. The investigators report that the use of vibrotactile PT significantly reduced the AHI at follow-up compared with baseline (mean difference (95% confidence interval [CI]) −9.19 events/hour [−11.68 to −6.70]; $P < .00001$). The mean percentage time spent in supine position (% supine TST) was also significantly reduced (mean difference (95% CI) −32.79% (−38.75% to −26.83%); $P < .00001$). The percentage changes in the AHI and % supine TST were 43% and 70%, respectively. Secondary outcomes were daytime sleepiness, quality of life, and sleep indices. These showed minimal change, although follow-up was short.[40] Similar results in comparison with a meta-analysis were published in 2017. Combined data for studies reporting on the effect of vibrotactile PT show that there was a mean AHI difference of 11.3 events/h (54% reduction) AHI and 33.6% (84% reduction) total sleeping time in the supine position. The standardized mean difference for both parameters demonstrated a large magnitude of effect (>0.8 in both cases).[35]

The effectiveness of PT is closely linked to patient compliance with the prescribed treatment regimen, which influences the total duration of treatment application throughout the night when obstructive events are prone to occur. The efficacy of treatment, in turn, signifies the treatment's capability to prevent obstructive respiratory events when physically applied. Effectiveness in clinical practice necessitates the fusion of both efficacy and compliance.[41] Therefore, when interpreting the results of conservative treatment approaches, it is paramount to recognize that the therapeutic effectiveness of a treatment is contingent not only on its impact on UA obstruction but also on the patient's adherence to the treatment protocol.[41–47] Mathematical formulas have been devised to quantify therapeutic effectiveness, and these calculations have been integrated into the literature.[41–47]

The tangible influence of compliance on the effectiveness of PT is vividly portrayed in an RCT involving 55 patients. The study's investigators concluded that both vibrotactile PT and TBT effectively reduced respiratory indices and minimized time spent in the supine sleep position to a median of 0%.[48] Notably, treatment success, defined as a reduction in the AHI to less than 5 events per hour, was achieved in 68.0% of the new-generation PT group and 42.9% of the TBT group ($P=.87$). However, compliance, characterized by adherence of at least 4 hours per night and at least 5 nights per week, was significantly higher among new-generation PT users, at 75.9%, in comparison to TBT users, at 42.3% ($P=.01$). This resulted in a mean alleviation of the disease of 48.6% and 70.5% for TBT and new-generation PT, respectively ($P=.005$). The mean disease alleviation is an indicator of therapeutic effectiveness, calculated as the product of adjusted compliance (PT use divided by total sleep time) with therapy efficacy (baseline AHI minus AHI with PT, expressed as a percentage), divided by 100.[45,49]

Objective measures of sleep quality and the frequency of awakenings exhibited more significant improvements in the vibrotactile PT group, as did the scores on the

Quebec Sleep Questionnaire.[48] The primary reasons for poor compliance with TBT, both in the short term (40%–70%) and long term (10%), encompass issues such as discomfort, back complaints, deterioration of sleep quality, and a lack of improvement in symptoms.[38,50–52]

In the case of vibrotactile PT, compliance is remarkably high under short-term study conditions (1 month), with median compliance percentages ranging from 76% to 96% when defined as 4 hours per night for 7 nights per week.[39,48,53] For those patients who continue to use the device over the long term (6–12 months), compliance remains high, ranging from 75% to 84.5% when defined as 4 hours per night for 7 nights per week.[54–56] Median hours of device use per night range from 5.2 to 5.5.[54,57] Beyers and colleagues[55] reported an average of 68.6 ± 25.6% of days of Sleep Position Trainer (SPT) use per week and an average SPT use of 7.3 ± 0.9 hours per night. In a prospective multicenter RCT comparing siOSA patients treated with SPT or auto-adjusting continuous positive airway pressure (aCPAP), the study concluded that treatment with SPT yielded non-inferior treatment efficacy and greater adherence to aCPAP.[58]

A third type of vibrotactile PT has been described in the literature. An eye mask SPT device composed of an eye mask and a forehead band, a snoring sensor, and a 3-axis gyro position sensor. The 3-axis gyro sensor in the middle of the SPT device is used to monitor changes in body position. A high-sensitivity snoring monitor is located on the side of the SPT device. A blood oxygen–monitoring accessory continuously monitors blood oxygen levels and the pulse rate. If the snoring sound exceeds 30 dB or the blood oxygen level drops below 85% for more than 3 seconds, the SPT device emits a low-frequency vibration to prompt the subject to change position.[59] The investigators performed an RCT, comparing the SPT eye mask, an oral device, and combination treatment with both devices. The rates of effective treatment in the SPT, oral appliance therapy, and combination therapy groups were 36.84%, 45%, and 80%, respectively, at month 6. Combination therapy has been been shown to result in higher therapeutic efficacy when compared to 1 of the treatment modalities alone.[60]

If the device is triggered by head position, it could be of particular interest for patients with POSA dependent solely on the position of the head. Furthermore, as reported in a study by van Kesteren and colleagues[22], in 46.2% of trunk supine position–dependent patients, head position was of considerable influence on the AHI (AHI was>5 higher when the head was also in supine position compared to when the head was turned to the side).

WHO ARE SUITABLE CANDIDATES?

Patients who are suitable for PT are those that will specifically benefit from a clinically significant improvement of their OSA with PT. siOSA patients could theoretically be cured by PT alone, whilst spOSA patients may need combination therapy. Other factors besides the AHI/respiratory disturbances to consider include time spent in the supine position.[61] When considering PT for PPs, one must take into account the following:

1. Insufficient distribution of various sleeping positions: Patients may not sleep in a certain position long enough for the AHI measured in that position to be valid and representative. Bignold and colleagues[14] mention a specific cut-off value of 20 minutes in a particular patient to be meaningful, whilst Ravesloot and colleagues[61] suggest 10% of the total sleep time.
2. Certain patients may “self-correct” their position to nonsupine sleep, and although they are known to have POSA, the treatment effect of PT might be limited.[62]

3. The preferred habitual sleeping position: Studies suggest that wearing a PSG apparatus leads to an increase in percentage of supine sleeping position causing an overestimation of OSA severity, especially in patients with POSA. This can have significant impact in both clinical and scientific practice.[63,64] Bearing this in mind, it is important to ask both the patient and partner, if applicable, what their preferred sleeping position is at home.
4. Chronic pain: Some patients are unable to sleep on their side. Reasons include shoulder or hip complaints and/or back pain in patients with ankylosing spondylitis and habitual prone sleepers using continuous positive airway pressure.

Another important element to consider is the subjective complaint of the patient. For example, if the patient's primary complaint is snoring in all sleeping positions, the patient (and potential partner) may not be pleased with the impact of PT on his/her main complaint even if it improves severity of POSA.

On a side and final note, PT is not only reserved for habitual snoring and POSA in adults. It has also been described in the literature as a treatment modality for patients with sleep paralysis and a floppy epiglottis as observed during drug-induced sleep endoscopy.[65,66] Sleep position has also been described as a potentially negative effect on the fetus resulting in altered growth, gestational length, and even death in maternal sleep.[67] Last but not least, there are also studies suggesting the use of PT in pediatric OSA patients.[68]

SUMMARY

POSA is a subtype of OSA in which the severity of the condition is primarily influenced by the patient's sleeping position. Compliance with PT, aimed at avoiding the supine sleep position, is crucial for its effectiveness. New-generation vibrotactile PT devices exhibit higher compliance rates and greater disease alleviation compared to traditional methods like the TBT. Recognizing the interplay between sleep position and disease severity is essential for personalized treatment strategies. The patient's comfort and adherence with PT, as well as an understanding of the relationship between sleep position and OSA severity are integral components of successful POSA management.

CLINICS CARE POINTS FOR POSITIONAL THERAPY IN OBSTRUCTIVE SLEEP APNEA

Pearls

- Consider POSA as a distinct subtype of OSA, whereby the severity of the condition is significantly influenced by the patient's sleeping position.
- Recognize that avoidance of the supine sleep position is a valuable therapeutic option for POSA management, as this position often exacerbates obstructive events.
- Choose your candidates wisely. Will they benefit from PT? Do they sleep on their back at home?
- Individualize treatment regimens, especially when using PT, to accommodate the unique needs and preferences of patients.
- Emphasize the importance of patient compliance with PT, as it plays a crucial role in the effectiveness of treatment, influencing both treatment success and disease alleviation.
- Stay updated with the latest advancements in PT, such as new-generation vibrotactile PT devices, which have shown higher compliance rates and greater disease alleviation compared to traditional methods like the TBT.

Pitfalls

- Avoid relying solely on PT for OSA management, as it may not be effective for all patients, and comorbid factors should be considered.

- Be cautious of the variable success and patient comfort associated with traditional PT methods like the TBT.
- Ensure proper patient education and follow-up to monitor compliance with PT, as poor adherence can diminish treatment effectiveness.
- Recognize that the relationship between sleep position and disease severity varies among patients, and PT may not be a one-size-fits-all solution.
- Remember that PT primarily targets the positional component of OSA and may not address anatomic or non-positional contributors to the condition.

DISCLOSURE

The author has no other funding, financial relationships, or conflicts of interest to disclose. M.J.L. Ravesloot is an investigator of Inspire.

REFERENCES

1. Taranto-Montemurro L, Messineo L, Wellman A. Targeting endotypic traits with medications for the pharmacological treatment of obstructive sleep apnea. A review of the current literature. J Clin Med 2019;8(11):1846.
2. Edwards BA, Redline S, Sands SA, et al. More than the sum of the respiratory events: personalized medicine approaches for obstructive sleep apnea. Am J Respir Crit Care Med 2019;200(6):691–703.
3. Eckert DJ, White DP, Jordan AS, et al. Defining phenotypic causes of obstructive sleep apnea. Identification of novel therapeutic targets. Am J Respir Crit Care Med 2013;188(8):996–1004.
4. Eckert DJ. Phenotypic approaches to positional therapy for obstructive sleep apnoea. Sleep Med Rev 2018;37:175–6.
5. Oksenberg A, Gadoth N. Positional patients (PP) and non positional patients (NPP) are two dominant phenotypes that should be included in the phenotypic approaches to obstructive sleep apnea. Sleep Med Rev 2018;37:173–4.
6. Ravesloot MJ, Frank MH, van Maanen JP, et al. Positional OSA part 2: retrospective cohort analysis with a new classification system (APOC). Sleep Breath 2015. https://doi.org/10.1007/s11325-015-1206-y.
7. Oksenberg A, Silverberg DS, Arons E, et al. Positional vs nonpositional obstructive sleep apnea patients: anthropomorphic, nocturnal polysomnographic, and multiple sleep latency test data. Chest 1997;112(3):629–39.
8. Richard W, Kox D, den Herder C, et al. The role of sleep position in obstructive sleep apnea syndrome. Eur Arch Oto-Rhino-Laryngol 2006;263(10):946–50.
9. Mador MJ, Kufel TJ, Magalang UJ, et al. Prevalence of positional sleep apnea in patients undergoing polysomnography. Chest 2005;128(4):2130–7.
10. Ravesloot M, Vonk P, Maurer J, et al. Standardized framework to report on the role of sleeping position in sleep apnea patients. Sleep Breath 2021;25:1717–28.
11. Oksenberg A, Gadoth N, Töyräs J, et al. Prevalence and characteristics of positional obstructive sleep apnea (POSA) in patients with severe OSA. Sleep Breath 2020;24:551–9.
12. Oksenberg A, Khamaysi I, Silverberg DS, et al. Association of body position with severity of apneic events in patients with severe nonpositional obstructive sleep apnea. Chest 2000;118(4):1018–24.
13. Cartwright RD. Effect of sleep position on sleep apnea severity. Sleep 1984;7(2):110–4.

14. Bignold JJ, Mercer JD, Antic NA, et al. Accurate position monitoring and improved supine-dependent obstructive sleep apnea with a new position recording and supine avoidance device. J Clin Sleep Med 2011;7(4):376–83.
15. Marklund M, Persson M, Franklin KA. Treatment success with a mandibular advancement device is related to supine-dependent sleep apnea. Chest 1998; 114(6):1630–5.
16. Permut I, Diaz-Abad M, Chatila W, et al. Comparison of positional therapy to CPAP in patients with positional obstructive sleep apnea. J Clin Sleep Med 2010;6(3):238–43.
17. Joosten SA, O'Donoghue FJ, Rochford PD, et al. Night-to-night repeatability of supine-related obstructive sleep apnea. Annals of the American Thoracic Society 2014;11(5):761–9.
18. Al Oweidat K, Toubasi AA, Montaha A-I, et al. Comparing the diagnostic value of the positional obstructive sleep apnea definitions. Respir Med 2023;212:107227.
19. Heinzer R, Petitpierre NJ, Marti-Soler H, Haba-Rubio J. Prevalence and characteristics of positional sleep apnea in the HypnoLaus population-based cohort. Sleep Med 2018;48:157–62.
20. Kim KT, Cho YW, Kim DE, et al. Two subtypes of positional obstructive sleep apnea: Supine-predominant and supine-isolated. Clin Neurophysiol 2016;127(1): 565–70.
21. Duce B, Kulkas A, Langton C, et al. Amsterdam positional OSA classification: the AASM 2012 recommended hypopnoea criteria increases the number of positional therapy candidates. Sleep Breath 2017;21(2):411–7.
22. van Kesteren ER, van Maanen JP, Hilgevoord AA, et al. Quantitative effects of trunk and head position on the apnea hypopnea index in obstructive sleep apnea. Sleep 2011;34(8):1075–81.
23. Walsh JH, Maddison KJ, Platt PR, et al. Influence of head extension, flexion, and rotation on collapsibility of the passive upper airway. Sleep 2008;31(10):1440–7.
24. Benoist L, Vonk P, de Vries N, et al. New-generation positional therapy in patients with positional central sleep apnea. European Archives of Oto-Rhino-Laryngology 2019;1–9.
25. Janssen H, Verbraecken JA, Pevernagie D, et al. Positional central sleep apnea. Positional therapy in obstructive sleep apnea 2015;209–19.
26. Oksenberg A, Arons E, Snir D, et al. Cheyne-Stokes respiration during sleep: a possible effect of body position. Med Sci Mon Int Med J Exp Clin Res 2002; 8(7):CS61–5.
27. Sahlin C, Svanborg E, Stenlund H, et al. Cheyne-Stokes respiration and supine dependency. Eur Respir J 2005;25(5):829–33.
28. Soll BA, Yeo KK, Davis JW, et al. The effect of posture on Cheyne-Stokes respirations and hemodynamics in patients with heart failure. Sleep 2009;32(11): 1499–507.
29. Szollosi I, Roebuck T, Thompson B, et al. Lateral sleeping position reduces severity of central sleep apnea/Cheyne-Stokes respiration. Sleep 2006;29(8): 1045–51.
30. Itasaka Y, Miyazaki S, Ishikawa K, et al. The influence of sleep position and obesity on sleep apnea. Psychiatry Clin Neurosci 2000;54(3):340–1.
31. Ann L, Lee C-H, Immen R, et al. Older Age is Associated with Positional Obstructive Sleep Apnea. Am J Geriatr Psychiatr 2023.
32. Mo JH, Lee CH, Rhee CS, et al. Positional dependency in Asian patients with obstructive sleep apnea and its implication for hypertension. Arch Otolaryngol Head Neck Surg 2011;137(8):786–90.

33. Tanaka F, Nakano H, Fau - Sudo N, et al. Relationship between the body position-specific apnea-hypopnea index and subjective sleepiness. (1423-0356 (Electronic)).
34. Teerapraipruk B, Chirakalwasan N, Simon R, et al. Clinical and polysomnographic data of positional sleep apnea and its predictors. Sleep Breath 2012;16:1167–72.
35. Ravesloot MJ, White D, Heinzer R, et al. Efficacy of the new generation of devices for positional therapy for patients with positional obstructive sleep apnea: a systematic review of the literature and meta-analysis. J Clin Sleep Med 2017;13(06): 813–24.
36. Barnes H, Edwards BA, Joosten SA, et al. Positional modification techniques for supine obstructive sleep apnea: a systematic review and meta-analysis. Sleep Med Rev 2017;36:107–15.
37. Rozanski JJ, Kleinfeld M. Patient's wife cures his snoring. Chest 1984;85(4):582.
38. Ravesloot MJ, van Maanen JP, Dun L, et al. The undervalued potential of positional therapy in position-dependent snoring and obstructive sleep apnea-a review of the literature. Sleep Breath 2013;17(1):39–49.
39. Levendowski DJ, Seagraves S, Popovic D, et al. Assessment of a neck-based treatment and monitoring device for positional obstructive sleep apnea. J Clin Sleep Med 2014;10(8):863–71.
40. ALQarni AS, Turnbull CD, Morrell MJ, et al. Efficacy of vibrotactile positional therapy devices on patients with positional obstructive sleep apnoea: a systematic review and meta-analysis. Thorax 2023.
41. Sutherland K, Phillips CL, Cistulli PA. Efficacy versus effectiveness in the treatment of obstructive sleep apnea: CPAP and oral appliances. Journal of Dental Sleep Medicine 2015;2(4):175–81.
42. Ravesloot MJ, de Vries N. Reliable calculation of the efficacy of non-surgical and surgical treatment of obstructive sleep apnea revisited. Sleep 2011;34(1):105–10.
43. Ravesloot MJ, de Vries N, Stuck BA. Treatment adherence should be taken into account when reporting treatment outcomes in obstructive sleep apnea. Laryngoscope 2014;124(1):344–5.
44. Stuck BA, Leitzbach S, Maurer JT. Effects of continuous positive airway pressure on apnea–hypopnea index in obstructive sleep apnea based on long-term compliance. Sleep Breath 2012;16:467–71.
45. Vanderveken OM, Dieltjens M, Wouters K, et al. Objective measurement of compliance during oral appliance therapy for sleep-disordered breathing. Thorax 2012. thoraxjnl-2012-201900.
46. Boyd SB, Walters AS. Effectiveness of treatment apnea-hypopnea index: a mathematical estimate of the true apnea-hypopnea index in the home setting. J Oral Maxillofac Surg 2013;71(2):351–7.
47. Bianchi MT, Alameddine Y, Mojica J. Apnea burden: efficacy versus effectiveness in patients using positive airway pressure. Sleep Med 2014;15(12):1579–81.
48. Eijsvogel MM, Ubbink R, Dekker J, et al. Sleep position trainer versus tennis ball technique in positional obstructive sleep apnea syndrome. J Clin Sleep Med 2015;11(2):139–47.
49. Grote L, Hedner J, Grunstein R, et al. Therapy with nCPAP: incomplete elimination of sleep related breathing disorder. Eur Respir J 2000;16(5):921–7.
50. Bignold JJ, Deans-Costi G, Goldsworthy MR, et al. Poor long-term patient compliance with the tennis ball technique for treating positional obstructive sleep apnea. J Clin Sleep Med 2009;5(5):428–30.
51. Heinzer RC, Pellaton C, Rey V, et al. Positional therapy for obstructive sleep apnea: an objective measurement of patients' usage and efficacy at home. Sleep Med 2012;13(4):425–8.

52. Oksenberg A, Silverberg D, Offenbach D, et al. Positional therapy for obstructive sleep apnea patients: A 6-month follow-up study. Laryngoscope 2006;116(11): 1995–2000.
53. van Maanen JP, Meester KA, Dun LN, et al. The sleep position trainer: a new treatment for positional obstructive sleep apnoea. Sleep Breath 2013;17(2):771–9.
54. de Ruiter MH, Benoist LB, De Vries N, et al. Durability of treatment effects of the Sleep Position Trainer versus oral appliance therapy in positional OSA: 12-month follow-up of a randomized controlled trial. Sleep Breath 2018;22:441–50.
55. Beyers J, Dieltjens M, Kastoer C, et al. Treatment of sleep-disordered breathing with positional therapy: long-term results. Eur Respiratory Soc 2019;23(4): 1141–9.
56. Laub RR, Tønnesen P, Jennum PJ. A Sleep Position Trainer for positional sleep apnea: a randomized, controlled trial. J Sleep Res 2017;26(5):641–50.
57. van Maanen JP, de Vries N. Long-term effectiveness and compliance of positional therapy with the sleep position trainer in the treatment of positional obstructive sleep apnea syndrome. Sleep 2014;37(7):1209–15.
58. Berry RB, Uhles ML, Abaluck BK, et al. NightBalance sleep position treatment device versus auto-adjusting positive airway pressure for treatment of positional obstructive sleep apnea. J Clin Sleep Med 2019;15(7):947–56.
59. Huang W, Li C, Zou J, et al. Effects of the combination of novel eye mask sleep position therapy device and oral appliance on positional OSA: A multi-arm, parallel-group randomized controlled trial. Sleep Med 2023;102:52–63.
60. Dieltjens M, Vroegop AV, Verbruggen AE, et al. A promising concept of combination therapy for positional obstructive sleep apnea. Sleep Breath 2015;19(2): 637–44.
61. Ravesloot M, Frank MH, van Maanen JP, et al. Towards a clinical classification system for position-dependent obstructive sleep apnea. Positional Therapy In Obstructive Sleep Apnea 2015;131–5.
62. Kaur A, Verma R, Gandhi A, et al. 0631 Effect of disease severity on determining body position during sleep in patients with positional obstructive sleep apnea. Sleep 2017;40(suppl_1):A233.
63. Vonk P, De Vries N, Ravesloot M. Polysomnography and sleep position, a Heisenberg phenomenon?: A large-scale series. HNO 2019;67(9):679–84.
64. Cerritelli L, Caranti A, Migliorelli A, et al. Sleep position and obstructive sleep apnea (OSA): Do we know how we sleep? A new explorative sleeping questionnaire. Sleep Breath 2022;26(4):1973–81.
65. Cui N, van Looij MA, Kasius KM. Successful treatment of sleep paralysis with the Sleep Position Trainer: a case report. J Clin Sleep Med 2022;18(9):2317–9.
66. Vonk P, Ravesloot M, Kasius K, et al. Floppy epiglottis during drug-induced sleep endoscopy: an almost complete resolution by adopting the lateral posture. Sleep Breath 2020;24:103–9.
67. Warland J, Dorrian J, Morrison JL, et al. Maternal sleep during pregnancy and poor fetal outcomes: a scoping review of the literature with meta-analysis. Sleep Med Rev 2018;41:197–219.
68. Xiao L, Baker A, Voutsas G, et al. Positional device therapy for the treatment of positional obstructive sleep apnea in children: a pilot study. Sleep Med 2021; 85:313–6.

Treatment of the Nose for Patients with Sleep Apnea

Jacquelyn K. Callander, MD, Jolie L. Chang, MD*

KEYWORDS

- Nasal obstruction • Nasal surgery • Obstructive sleep apnea • CPAP compliance
- Sleep-disordered breathing

KEY POINTS

- Patients with obstructive sleep apnea (OSA) frequently experience nasal obstruction. Clinical evaluation of patients with OSA should include a history of nasal obstruction symptoms and a detailed examination of the nose.
- Patients with nasal obstruction are at higher risk of continuous positive airway pressure (CPAP) intolerance, and in this population, nasal surgery helps to improve CPAP tolerance if nasal obstruction is the main subjective barrier to use.
- Treatment of nasal obstruction via intranasal corticosteroids may improve subjective daytime sleepiness and is associated with a minimal decrease in OSA severity.
- In children, adenotonsillectomy is the primary surgical therapy for moderate to severe OSA or mild OSA that does not respond to intranasal corticosteroids, but turbinate reduction should be considered in those with concomitant severe allergic rhinitis or persistent OSA.
- Nasal surgery improves subjective daytime sleepiness in patients with OSA and nasal obstruction, although it is unlikely to result in a meaningful reduction in OSA severity.

INTRODUCTION

Obstructive sleep apnea (OSA) is characterized by reduction or cessation of airflow during sleep due to upper airway collapse. The involvement of the nasal cavity and nasopharynx in this disease state has long been a subject of debate. In 1861, George Caitlin published "The Breath of Life," which proposed that the root cause of sleep-related health issues lay in mouth breathing.[1] Over a century and a half later, mouth taping during sleep became a viral sensation on social media platforms, with claims of increased energy and mood.[2] Investigation into the role of the nasal airway in OSA began late in the twentieth century. Early studies evaluated the effects of artificial nasal obstruction via placement of packing, which was shown to worsen polysomnographic variables

Department of Otolaryngology-Head & Neck Surgery, University of California, San Francisco, CA, USA
* Corresponding author. 2233 Post St 3rd Floor, San Francisco, CA 94115.
E-mail address: Jolie.Chang@ucsf.edu

Otolaryngol Clin N Am 57 (2024) 491–500
https://doi.org/10.1016/j.otc.2023.11.002
0030-6665/24/Published by Elsevier Inc.

in patients with sleep-disordered breathing (SDB) and even induce apneas and hypopneas to variable degrees in healthy subjects.[3,4] In 1997, the first population-based study was published with nearly 5000 subjects surveyed, and an association was found between nasal obstruction symptoms and symptoms of SDB.[5]

This article explores the following questions.

1. What is the relationship of nasal obstruction and OSA—are they merely comorbid or is there a causative role?
2. How does treatment of nasal obstruction affect patients with OSA?
3. Which OSA patients will benefit most from treatment of nasal obstruction?

EPIDEMIOLOGY

Owing to the high prevalence of both OSA and nasal obstruction, these conditions are often comorbid but the impact of each one on the other remains controversial. Nasal pathologies contributing to chronic obstruction can be grouped by (1) anatomic abnormalities including septal deviation, nasal valve incompetence, and craniofacial anomalies and (2) inflammatory disorders including allergic or nonallergic rhinitis, chronic rhinosinusitis with or without polyps, and other pathologies. The prevalence of nasal obstruction is difficult to calculate because many diagnoses are associated with nasal obstruction and individuals may not seek formal medical care for nasal obstruction, but the median worldwide estimate of unspecified rhinitis alone is 29.4%.[6] Data from the Icelandic Sleep Apnea Cohort suggest that 35% of OSA patients experience nocturnal nasal obstruction ≥3 times per week before initiating treatment with continuous positive airway pressure (CPAP), and this subgroup reports more daytime sleepiness.[7] Compared with healthy controls, patients with OSA also demonstrate higher baseline scores for measures of sinonasal disease based on a visual analog scale and the sinonasal outcome test-20.[8]

THE RELATIONSHIP BETWEEN NASAL OBSTRUCTION AND OBSTRUCTIVE SLEEP APNEA: WHAT IS THE PATHOPHYSIOLOGIC BASIS?

The nasal airway accounts for more than 50% of total airway resistance.[9] Recumbent posture during sleep increases venous engorgement within the nose leading to more nasal resistance and decreased airflow, a phenomenon intensified in patients with baseline congestion.[10] Although most studies have found no association between nasal resistance and OSA, several studies have shown correlation between nasal resistance or nasal volume and apnea-hypopnea index (AHI) and oxygen desaturation index (ODI). Virkkula and colleagues demonstrated this effect to be greater in nonobese subjects.[11] In addition, a study of 541 snorers showed nasal resistance contributed to 2.3% of the AHI variance, with body mass index (BMI), sex, age, and mandibular plane-hyoid distance as factors contributing more significantly to the AHI.[12] Other aspects of nasal anatomy (turbinate hypertrophy, presence of septal deviation, and nasal valve collapse) have been studied without demonstrating correlation to OSA.[13] Thus, the impact of nasal obstruction on the pathophysiology of OSA remains controversial and results emphasize a complex interplay of contributing factors.

PHYSIOLOGIC NASAL-RELATED CONTRIBUTORS TO OBSTRUCTIVE SLEEP APNEA

Nasal Sensory Input

Correlation between objective nasal resistance and subjective reports of nasal obstruction is poor.[14] The same degree of septal deviation or turbinate hypertrophy causing bothersome symptoms in one patient may be asymptomatic in the next. Subjective nasal patency has been linked to a thermoreceptor activated by nasal mucosal cooling; thus, patency is more significantly correlated to the dynamic change of nasal mucosal temperature than airflow resistance.[15] This same phenomenon may be at play in OSA. Activation of nasal thermoreceptors via cold air increases genioglossus muscle activity; this is reversed with topical nasal anesthesia. Similarly, topical nasal anesthesia alone induces apneas and hypopneas in subjects who demonstrate normal AHI under placebo conditions.[16]

Mouth Breathing

It has been speculated that increased nasal resistance or decrease nasal volume may shift the breathing route from nasal to oral, and the threshold of obstruction that prompts this shift varies between individuals. Mouth breathing, which has been defined as greater than 30% of airflow through the oral cavity, has been linked to a variety of maladaptations, as it leads to posterior displacement of the jaw and subsequent increase in upper airway obstruction at the tongue base and lateral pharynx during sleep.[17] Upper airway resistance during sleep is up to 2.5 times higher while breathing orally versus nasally.[17] However, mouth breathing is common in OSA independent of nasal obstruction, and some patients may continue to mouth breathe even after nasal obstruction is reversed.

Downstream Upper Airway Anatomy

The Starling resistor model describes the upper airway as a collapsible tube bound on either end by fixed segments (nasal passage and trachea).[18] When resistance is increased in the nasal passage, the lungs must generate additional negative pressure to maintain stable airflows, thereby causing increased risk for collapse of the pliable pharyngeal segment.[18] Real-life anatomy is undoubtedly more complex than this model, with many factors that could influence collapse of the pharynx.

THE NASAL AIRWAY AND CONTINUOUS POSITIVE AIRWAY PRESSURE COMPLIANCE

CPAP remains a first-line therapy to treat moderate to severe OSA. Despite its potential to reduce AHI and improve symptoms, the overall efficacy of this therapeutic option is limited by variable individual compliance. Many factors have been shown to influence patient compliance with CPAP, including severity of OSA, perceived benefit of therapy, inconvenience, discomfort, and claustrophobia wearing a mask.[19] Nasal problems with CPAP are commonly reported, including obstruction, rhinorrhea, sneezing, and dryness.

Several studies have linked objective measures of nasal anatomy with CPAP compliance. Sugiura and colleagues found that nasal resistance measured by rhinomanometry before CPAP initiation predicted CPAP acceptance, with higher resistance predicting lower acceptance rates.[20] The nasal minimal cross-sectional area and nasal volumes, which were not correlated to subjective nasal congestion, predicted CPAP use.[21] Park and colleagues demonstrated that higher severity of septal deviation and turbinate hypertrophy is associated with worse CPAP adherence.[19]

The assessment of nasal symptoms is more clinically meaningful, as the use of rhinomanometry or acoustic rhinometry is not a regular part of clinical practice. Haddad and colleagues found that lower or better nasal symptom scores were associated with increased CPAP use.[22] Another study of concurrent rhinitis and OSA demonstrated an inverse relationship between CPAP compliance and nasal symptom scores.[23] A prospective cohort study of 147 subjects with newly diagnosed OSA identified subjective nasal congestion as an independent predictor of poor CPAP compliance.[24]

THE ROLE OF MEDICAL THERAPIES FOR NASAL OBSTRUCTION AND IMPACT ON OBSTRUCTIVE SLEEP APNEA

Nasal Steroids

Several randomized controlled trials (RCTs) nonspecific to OSA demonstrated improved subjective daytime sleepiness in patients with allergic rhinitis after consistent use of intranasal steroids (INSs).[25] An RCT of 23 snorers with allergic rhinitis treated with fluticasone and placebo in a crossover 4-week study demonstrated a significant improvement in AHI by a median of 6.5 events/hour in the OSA group.[26] A systematic review and meta-analysis evaluating the effect of INSs on CPAP use included three randomized clinical controlled trials ($N = 224$) and identified a pooled difference of 27 minutes/night of CPAP use with fluticasone versus placebo, which did not meet statistical significance.[27] Overall, the literature suggests that INS use has a small positive therapeutic impact on OSA in patients with concomitant rhinitis.

Antihistamines

An RCT of 80 patients with OSA and allergic rhinitis evaluated the effect of nasal steroids with or without an oral antihistamine revealing a significant improvement in posttreatment AHI and Epworth Sleepiness Scale (ESS) scores in the nasal steroid group + placebo as well as the nasal steroid + antihistamine group, without significant differences between groups. The investigators concluded that INSs show significant benefit, but oral antihistamines do not.[28] No studies thus far have specifically evaluated nasal antihistamine use alone and its effect on OSA. However, in patients with concomitant allergic rhinitis, it may be reasonable to add antihistamine to an INS for optimal benefit, without the expectation that a nasal antihistamine alone would improve objective measures of OSA.[25]

Nasal Dilators

The only meta-analysis evaluated 14 studies on internal nasal dilators and external nasal dilator strips in 114 subjects with OSA. This showed no significant change in AHI, oxygen saturation nadir, or daytime sleepiness.[29] Although nasal dilators do not effectively improve objective measures of OSA, they may play a role in decreasing CPAP pressure which could improve adherence, though pressure reduction is modest and significant only in patients requiring pressures above 9 cm H_2O.[30,31]

Medical Therapies to Treat the Nose in Pediatric Obstructive Sleep Apnea

In the pediatric population, nasal steroids are uniquely aimed at reducing adenoid hypertrophy. A double-blind placebo-controlled study of 62 children with confirmed mild OSA showed a small but significant improvement in AHI and ODI in patients treated with intranasal mometasone versus placebo.[32] Of note, a double-blind RCT comparing 6 weeks of intranasal mometasone to nasal saline in 276 children found no difference between groups in rate of symptomatic improvement; however, 44% (95% CI 36%–53%) of the NS group and 41% (95% CI 32%–49%) of the saline group reported resolution of SDB symptoms.[33] This study suggests that in children, it is reasonable to trial either a nasal steroid or nasal saline during treatment for SDB.

Montelukast is a leukotriene antagonist widely used in children with OSA, as this class of medications is thought to decrease the size of adenotonsillar tissue by targeting proliferation pathways.[34] A systematic review identified five studies ($N = 166$) evaluating montelukast monotherapy and demonstrated a 56% improvement in AHI (6.2 ± 3.1 events/hour pretreatment and 2.7 ± 2.7 events/hour posttreatment).[35] Two additional studies ($N = 502$) of combined treatment with NS and oral montelukast showed an even greater treatment effect of 70% improvement in AHI (4.8 ± 2.1

events/hour to 1.4 ± 0.4 events/hour post-treatment).[35] Despite evidence of efficacy in the pediatric population, montelukast has fallen out of favor after a black box warning was issued in 2020 by the Food and Drug Administration due to a low but present risk for increased neuropsychiatric events, including suicidal thoughts.[36]

In pediatric patients with mild OSA, an initial trial of medical therapy with INS can be considered before adenotonsillectomy. The addition of oral montelukast is reasonable, but the potential adverse effects should be discussed thoroughly with parents.

THE ROLE OF NASAL SURGERY TO ADDRESS MEASURES OF OBSTRUCTIVE SLEEP APNEA

Nasal Surgery to Address Objective Measures of Obstructive Sleep Apnea

Surgical interventions to address nasal obstruction include septoplasty, turbinate reduction, functional rhinoplasty, and sinus surgery. One RCT compared isolated septoplasty to sham surgery in patients with OSA.[37] The investigators found no significant decrease in AHI in a majority of the surgery group, though 4 of 27 (12.8%) met criteria for success, defined as postoperative AHI less than 15 events/hour and ≥50% decrease from the baseline AHI.[37] In the most recent systematic review on the topic by Schoustra and colleagues, 21 relevant studies of isolated nasal surgery for the treatment of sleep apnea were identified.[38] Eighteen of these were feasible for meta-analysis of AHI, revealing a small overall decrease in AHI of 4.08 events/hour from preoperative to postoperative polysomnogram (PSG). This result reflected an earlier meta-analysis by Wu and colleagues, which included 18 studies with mean improvement in AHI of 4.15 events/hour ($P < .01$).[39] Overall, the data suggest a small decrease in AHI after isolated nasal surgery.

In children with persistent severe allergic rhinitis, the addition of inferior turbinate reduction to adenotonsillectomy resulted in decreased postoperative AHI (0.8 events/hour) as opposed to adenotonsillectomy alone (3.5 events/hour); AHI improvement after surgery was associated with decreased minimal nasal cross-sectional area.[40] In pediatric patients with turbinate hypertrophy who have previously undergone adenotonsillectomy but have persistent OSA, it is reasonable to consider turbinate reduction based on expert consensus statement from the American Academy of Otolaryngology-Head and Neck Surgery.[41]

Nasal Surgery to Address Subjective Measures of Obstructive Sleep Apnea

All meta-analyses of isolated nasal surgery to date demonstrated a significant improvement in ESS, with reported mean differences ranging from −4.08 to -3.5 points.[38,39,42,43] This is a critical finding, given AHI often does not align with subjective symptoms of OSA, and recent studies have demonstrated that patients with OSA and excessive daytime sleepiness are at a significantly higher risk for cardiovascular and metabolic disease.[44] Nasal surgery also leads to an improvement in self- and bed partner-reported snoring, though complete cessation of snoring after nasal surgery alone is uncommon.[42] In addition, patients with comorbid chronic rhinosinusitis and OSA demonstrate a significantly lower quality of life, and endoscopic sinus surgery has been shown to improve subjective sleep quality.[45]

There are strong data supporting the role of nasal surgery to improve CPAP tolerance.[38] An increase in nightly CPAP usage from 0.5 hours preoperatively to 5 hours postoperatively was shown in a small cohort (N = 18) of patients who reported nasal obstruction as the sole reason for intolerance.[46] Similarly, Elwany and colleagues reported 100% CPAP compliance (use of CPAP ≥ 4 hours on ≥ 70% of nights) and significantly decreased CPAP pressures after nasal surgery in 49 patients who were previously non-CPAP compliant solely due to nasal obstruction.[47] OSA patients were much more likely to transition from poor CPAP compliance to good CPAP compliance ($\geq$ 4 hours per night) if they reported nasal obstruction as the sole barrier to CPAP use preoperatively.[48] In a large population-based study, nasal polyposis was independently linked with CPAP usage of less than 4 hours per night, indicating that surgical and medical therapy to address chronic rhinosinusitis with nasal polyposis would lead to improved CPAP adherence.[49] The literature largely supports improvement in CPAP compliance after nasal surgery specifically in patients who report nasal obstruction as the sole barrier to use. Lower CPAP pressures requirements contributed to improved CPAP tolerance.

IS THERE A SUBSET OF OBSTRUCTIVE SLEEP APNEA PATIENTS WHO BENEFIT MOST FROM NASAL SURGERY?

Several patient-specific factors are likely to influence the efficacy of nasal surgery in the treatment of sleep apnea. Morinaga and colleagues evaluated the effect of pharyngeal morphology during awake examination on effectiveness of nasal surgery to treat sleep apnea, finding that a lower modified Mallampati score and wider retroglossal space predicted increased improvement in AHI after nasal surgery.[50] Similarly, Li and colleagues found that Friedman tongue position grades I or II correlated with decreased AHI after nasal surgery alone for OSA.[51] Kim and colleagues found significant reduction in AHI in cohort of patients undergoing isolated nasal surgery for sleep apnea, but this effect was much greater in the subgroup that had allergic rhinitis or moderate to severe nasal obstruction based on preoperative Nasal Obstruction Symptom Evaluation score.[52] Finally, lower BMI has been linked to improved outcomes after isolated nasal surgery for OSA.[51]

DISCUSSION

The relationship between nasal obstruction and OSA is complex. There are several pathophysiologic connections between nasal obstruction and OSA, including potential risk for increased pharyngeal collapse in a state of high nasal resistance, the increased likelihood of mouth breathing in the setting of nasal obstruction, and blunting of the nasal ventilatory reflex via decreased nasal airflow. The assessment of OSA outcomes after nasal surgery is plagued by heterogenous patient populations with varying severities and etiologies of OSA and nasal pathologies, inconsistent surgical methods and criteria for patient selection, and small sample sizes. This is compounded by the poor correlation between subjective symptoms of nasal obstruction and objective nasal resistance or volume. Literature supports medical management with steroid nasal sprays as first-line therapy in patients with OSA and nasal obstruction, as well as patients with CPAP noncompliance due to nasal obstruction. In medically refractory cases, studies suggest that a subset of individuals may benefit from nasal surgery alone, with potentially influential factors including lower BMI and preexisting nasal pathology. Additional research is warranted to better understand predictors for surgical success and OSA improvement. Nasal surgery also has a significant role in improving daytime sleepiness, though it is unlikely to cure moderate to severe OSA. Nasal surgery should be performed in patients with OSA with the goal of improvement of direct symptoms of nasal obstruction; however, in appropriate patients, it may also be viewed as an adjunct to improve tolerance of CPAP or as a component of multilevel surgery aimed at upper airway collapse. These recommendations are in line with the 2023 International Consensus Statement on OSA, which stresses that the decision to treat nasal obstruction in this patient population should be based on both clinical examination and shared-decision making surrounding goals of therapy.[31]

SUMMARY

The pathogenesis of OSA is multifactorial and requires an individualized approach tailored to each patient, a principle that holds true when considering the nasal airway. Nasal obstruction has a deleterious impact on objective and subjective measures of OSA and can lead to decreased CPAP compliance. Both medical and surgical management of nasal obstruction have demonstrated increased CPAP adherence, particularly in the subset of patients who report nasal obstruction as the main barrier to compliance. Treatment of OSA patients with comorbid rhinitis via topical nasal steroids has a beneficial impact on daytime sleepiness, though the effect on OSA severity is minimal. When nasal obstruction is not amenable to topical treatment, nasal surgery has been shown to result in decreased daytime sleepiness. Therefore, medical and surgical treatment of nasal obstruction should be regarded as adjunct treatments alongside more definitive measures to address downstream upper airway collapse in OSA.

CLINICS CARE POINTS

- Patients with obstructive sleep apnea (OSA) frequently experience nasal obstruction. Clinical evaluation of patients with obstructive sleep apnea should include a history of nasal obstruction symptoms and a detailed examination of the nose.
- Patients with nasal obstruction are at higher risk of continuous positive airway pressure (CPAP) intolerance, and in this population, nasal surgery may help improve CPAP tolerance if nasal obstruction is the main subjective barrier to use.
- Treatment of nasal obstruction via intranasal corticosteroids may improve subjective daytime sleepiness and is associated with a minimal decrease in OSA severity.
- Nasal surgery improves subjective daytime sleepiness in patients with OSA and nasal obstruction, although it is unlikely to result in a meaningful reduction in OSA severity.
- In children, adenotonsillectomy is the main surgical therapy for moderate to severe OSA or mild OSA that does not respond to intranasal corticosteroids, but turbinate reduction should be considered in those with concomitant severe allergic rhinitis or persistent OSA.
- Some OSA patients may benefit more from nasal surgery, including those with moderate to severe nasal obstruction, lower Friedman tongue position grade, and lower baseline BMI, but further research is needed to identify predictors of surgical success.

DISCLOSURE

The authors have no relevant disclosures.

REFERENCES

1. Caitlin G. The breath of life, or mal-respiration, and its effects upon the enjyments & life of man. New York, NY: John Wiley & Son Publishers; 1861.
2. Blum D. Can a piece of tape help you sleep?, 6. New York, NY: The New York Times; 2022.

3. Taasan V, Wynne JW, Cassisi N, et al. The effect of nasal packing on sleep-disordered breathing and nocturnal oxygen desaturation. Laryngoscope 1981;91(7):1163–72.
4. Olsen KD, Kern EB, Westbrook PR. Sleep and breathing disturbance secondary to nasal obstruction. Otolaryngol Head Neck Surg 1981;89(5):804–10.
5. Young T, Finn L, Kim H. Nasal obstruction as a risk factor for sleep-disordered breathing. The University of Wisconsin Sleep and Respiratory Research Group. J Allergy Clin Immunol 1997;99(2):S757–62.
6. Savouré M, Bousquet J, Jaakkola JJK, et al. Worldwide prevalence of rhinitis in adults: A review of definitions and temporal evolution. Clin Transl Allergy 2022;12(3):e12130.
7. Värendh M, Andersson M, Bjørnsdottir E, et al. Nocturnal nasal obstruction is frequent and reduces sleep quality in patients with obstructive sleep apnea. J Sleep Res 2018;27(4):e12631.
8. Moxness MHS, Bugten V, Thorstensen WM, et al. Sinonasal characteristics in patients with obstructive sleep apnea compared to healthy controls. Int J Otolaryngol 2017;2017:1935284.
9. Ferris BG Jr, Mead J, Opie LH. Partitioning of respiratory flow resistance in man. J Appl Physiol 1964;19:653–8.
10. Calvo-Henríquez C, Chiesa-Estomba C, Lechien JR, et al. The Recumbent Position Affects Nasal Resistance: A Systematic Review and Meta-Analysis. Laryngoscope 2022;132(1):6–16.
11. Virkkula P, Maasilta P, Hytönen M, et al. Nasal obstruction and sleep-disordered breathing: the effect of supine body position on nasal measurements in snorers. Acta Otolaryngol 2003;123(5):648–54.
12. Miljeteig H, Hoffstein V, Cole P. The effect of unilateral and bilateral nasal obstruction on snoring and sleep apnea. Laryngoscope 1992;102(10):1150–2.
13. Leitzen KP, Brietzke SE, Lindsay RW. Correlation between nasal anatomy and objective obstructive sleep apnea severity. Otolaryngol Head Neck Surg 2014;150(2):325–31.
14. Stewart MG, Smith TL. Objective versus subjective outcomes assessment in rhinology. Am J Rhinol 2005;19(5):529–35.
15. Zhao K, Jiang J, Blacker K, et al. Regional peak mucosal cooling predicts the perception of nasal patency. Laryngoscope 2014;124(3):589–95.
16. White DP, Cadieux RJ, Lombard RM, et al. The effects of nasal anesthesia on breathing during sleep. Am Rev Respir Dis 1985;132(5):972–5.
17. Fitzpatrick MF, McLean H, Urton AM, et al. Effect of nasal or oral breathing route on upper airway resistance during sleep. Eur Respir J 2003;22(5):827–32.
18. Smith PL, Wise RA, Gold AR, et al. Upper airway pressure-flow relationships in obstructive sleep apnea. J Appl Physiol (1985) 1988;64(2):789–95.
19. Park P, Kim J, Song YJ, et al. Influencing factors on CPAP adherence and anatomic characteristics of upper airway in OSA subjects. Medicine (Baltim) 2017;96(51):e8818.
20. Sugiura T, Noda A, Nakata S, et al. Influence of nasal resistance on initial acceptance of continuous positive airway pressure in treatment for obstructive sleep apnea syndrome. Respiration 2007;74(1):56–60.
21. Li HY, Engleman H, Hsu CY, et al. Acoustic reflection for nasal airway measurement in patients with obstructive sleep apnea-hypopnea syndrome. Sleep 2005;28(12):1554–9.

22. Haddad FL, Vidigal Tde A, Mello-Fujita L, et al. The influence of nasal abnormalities in adherence to continuous positive airway pressure device therapy in obstructive sleep apnea patients. Sleep Breath 2013;17(4):1201–7.
23. Parikh NG, Junaid I, Sheinkopf L, et al. Clinical control in the dual diagnosis of obstructive sleep apnea syndrome and rhinitis: a prospective analysis. Am J Rhinol Allergy 2014;28(1):e52–5.
24. Wu H, Fang F, Guo Y, et al. Independent role of nasal congestion in positive airway pressure compliance for OSA treatment. Otolaryngol Head Neck Surg 2022;167(2):395–402.
25. Ferguson BJ. Influences of allergic rhinitis on sleep. Otolaryngol Head Neck Surg 2004;130(5):617–29.
26. Kiely JL, Nolan P, McNicholas WT. Intranasal corticosteroid therapy for obstructive sleep apnoea in patients with co-existing rhinitis. Thorax 2004;59(1):50–5.
27. Charakorn N, Hirunwiwatkul P, Chirakalwasan N, et al. The effects of topical nasal steroids on continuous positive airway pressure compliance in patients with obstructive sleep apnea: a systematic review and meta-analysis. Sleep Breath 2017;21(1):3–8.
28. Acar M, Cingi C, Sakallioglu O, et al. The effects of mometasone furoate and desloratadine in obstructive sleep apnea syndrome patients with allergic rhinitis. Am J Rhinol Allergy 2013;27(4):e113–6.
29. Camacho M, Malu OO, Kram YA, et al. Nasal dilators (breathe right strips and nozovent) for snoring and OSA: a systematic review and meta-analysis. Pulm Med 2016;2016:4841310.
30. Schönhofer B, Kerl J, Suchi S, et al. Effect of nasal valve dilation on effective CPAP level in obstructive sleep apnea. Respir Med 2003;97(9):1001–5.
31. Chang JL, Goldberg AN, Alt JA, et al. International consensus statement on obstructive sleep apnea. Int Forum Allergy Rhinol 2023;13(7):1061–482.
32. Chan CC, Au CT, Lam HS, et al. Intranasal corticosteroids for mild childhood obstructive sleep apnea–a randomized, placebo-controlled study. Sleep Med 2015;16(3):358–63.
33. Baker A, Grobler A, Davies K, et al. Effectiveness of intranasal mometasone furoate vs saline for sleep-disordered breathing in children: a randomized clinical trial. JAMA Pediatr 2023;177(3):240–7.
34. Dayyat E, Serpero LD, Kheirandish-Gozal L, et al. Leukotriene pathways and in vitro adenotonsillar cell proliferation in children with obstructive sleep apnea. Chest 2009;135(5):1142–9.
35. Liming BJ, Ryan M, Mack D, et al. Montelukast and nasal corticosteroids to treat pediatric obstructive sleep apnea: a systematic review and meta-analysis. Otolaryngol Head Neck Surg 2019;160(4):594–602.
36. Paljarvi T, Forton J, Luciano S, et al. Analysis of Neuropsychiatric Diagnoses After Montelukast Initiation. JAMA Netw Open 2022;5(5):e2213643.
37. Koutsourelakis I, Georgoulopoulos G, Perraki E, et al. Randomised trial of nasal surgery for fixed nasal obstruction in obstructive sleep apnoea. Eur Respir J 2008;31(1):110–7.
38. Schoustra E, van Maanen P, den Haan C, et al. The role of isolated nasal surgery in obstructive sleep apnea therapy-a systematic review. Brain Sci 2022;12(11):1446.
39. Wu J, Zhao G, Li Y, et al. Apnea-hypopnea index decreased significantly after nasal surgery for obstructive sleep apnea: a meta-analysis. Medicine (Baltim) 2017;96(5):e6008.

40. Cheng PW, Fang KM, Su HW, et al. Improved objective outcomes and quality of life after adenotonsillectomy with inferior turbinate reduction in pediatric obstructive sleep apnea with inferior turbinate hypertrophy. Laryngoscope 2012;122(12):2850–4.
41. Ishman SL, Maturo S, Schwartz S, et al. Expert consensus statement: management of pediatric persistent obstructive sleep apnea after adenotonsillectomy. Otolaryngol Head Neck Surg 2023;168(2):115–30.
42. Li HY, Wang PC, Chen YP, et al. Critical appraisal and meta-analysis of nasal surgery for obstructive sleep apnea. Am J Rhinol Allergy 2011;25(1):45–9.
43. Ishii L, Roxbury C, Godoy A, et al. Does nasal surgery improve OSA in patients with nasal obstruction and OSA? a meta-analysis. Otolaryngol Head Neck Surg 2015;153(3):326–33.
44. Allen AJH, Jen R, Mazzotti DR, et al. Symptom subtypes and risk of incident cardiovascular and cerebrovascular disease in a clinic-based obstructive sleep apnea cohort. J Clin Sleep Med 2022;18(9):2093–102.
45. Sukato DC, Abramowitz JM, Boruk M, et al. Endoscopic sinus surgery improves sleep quality in chronic rhinosinusitis: a systematic review and meta-analysis. Otolaryngol Head Neck Surg 2018;158(2):249–56.
46. Poirier J, George C, Rotenberg B. The effect of nasal surgery on nasal continuous positive airway pressure compliance. Laryngoscope 2014;124(1):317–9.
47. Elwany S, Bahgat AY, Ibrahim M, et al. Surgical correction of nasal obstruction in obstructive sleep apnea improves CPAP outcomes and compliance. Ir J Med Sci 2022;191(6):2723–8.
48. Cha H, Oh H, Han SA, et al. The clinical influence of nasal surgery on PAP compliance and optimal application among OSA subjects uncomfortable with PAP device wear. Sci Rep 2023;13(1):4383.
49. Bengtsson C, Grote L, Ljunggren M, et al. Nasal polyposis is a risk factor for nonadherence to CPAP treatment in sleep apnea: the population-based DISCOVERY study. J Clin Sleep Med 2023;19(3):573–9.
50. Morinaga M, Nakata S, Yasuma F, et al. Pharyngeal morphology: a determinant of successful nasal surgery for sleep apnea. Laryngoscope 2009;119(5):1011–6.
51. Li HY, Lee LA, Wang PC, et al. Can nasal surgery improve obstructive sleep apnea: subjective or objective? Am J Rhinol Allergy 2009;23(6):e51–5.
52. Kim SD, Jung DW, Lee JW, et al. Relationship between allergic rhinitis and nasal surgery success in patients with obstructive sleep apnea. Am J Otolaryngol 2021;42(6):103079.

Advances in Pharyngeal Surgery Over the Past 10 Years: New Techniques and Technology

Stuart G. Mackay, MBBS, FRACS[a,b,c], James D. Every, MD, BMedSci[a,b,*]

KEYWORDS

- Pharyngeal surgery • Airway surgery • Obstructive sleep apnea • Surgical technique

KEY POINTS

- Advances in published literature have confirmed the role of pharyngeal surgery in salvage treatment of obstructive sleep apnea (OSA) in adults and as primary treatment of OSA in pediatrics.
- Advances in surgical technique and anatomic understanding are resulting in wider availability and effectiveness of multilevel airway surgery.
- Advances in assessment evaluate dynamic airway collapse in decision-making for OSA treatment.
- Advances in collaboration have explored mean disease alleviation, endo-phenotype outcomes, and the importance of multidisciplinary care in pharyngeal surgery for OSA.
- Achieving clinically important outcomes with pharyngeal surgery and mean disease alleviation opens debate for exploring the broader role of pharyngeal surgery in OSA.

This article is devoted to a review of advances in Pharyngeal Surgery over the past 10 years. Pharyngeal Surgery is defined herein as a cluster of operative interventions designed to open or stabilize the upper airway from nasopharynx to laryngopharynx, in adult and pediatric patients with obstructive sleep apnea/sleep-disordered breathing. Interventions from 2013 to current are included, provided they are published in the peer reviewed literature and generally accepted by the International Surgical Sleep Society community. Such surgeries have been tabulated in various publications in the last decade (eg, Table 1 in 2013 MJA Perspectives[1]).

[a] Department of Otolaryngology, Head and Neck Surgery, The Wollongong Hospital, Wollongong, New South Wales, Australia; [b] School of Medicine, University of Wollongong, Wollongong, New South Wales, Australia; [c] Illawarra ENT Head and Neck Clinic, 8-10 Victoria Street, Wollongong, New South Wales 2500, Australia
* Corresponding author. The Wollongong Hospital, Loftus Street, Wollongong, NSW 2500.
E-mail address: sgmackay@ozemail.com.au

Otolaryngol Clin N Am 57 (2024) 501–510
https://doi.org/10.1016/j.otc.2024.02.009 oto.theclinics.com

The pharyngeal surgeon involved in adult and pediatric OSA surgery has a primary focus on seeking high-benefit/low-risk interventions based on the highest level contemporary evidence. Indications for airway surgery may include the following:

1. Primary adenotonsillectomy in pediatric sleep breathing disorders
2. Poor compliance/tolerance of device therapy in adult OSA
3. Intolerable complications of device therapy in adult OSA
4. Salvage pediatric airway surgery for residual disease after prior adenotonsillectomy
5. Patient favors surgery, declining all other options, or patient has particularly favorable anatomy for surgery in adult OSA/snoring

The relevant advances in the last decade will be explored under the headings that follow:

1. Advances in Published Literature
2. Advances in Surgical Technique
3. Advances in Assessment
4. Advances in Collaboration
5. Future

ADVANCES IN PUBLISHED LITERATURE

Since 2013, several well-designed and executed randomized clinical trials in pharyngeal surgery have solidified the role of salvage OSA interventions in adults and primary OSA treatment in pediatrics. The most relevant of these are discussed in the this section.

Sleep Apnea Multilevel Surgery Trial—2020

The Sleep Apnea Multilevel Surgery (SAMS) randomized clinical trial evaluated multilevel pharyngeal surgery (modified uvulopalatopharyngoplasty [UPPP] and radiofrequency tongue channeling) in adults with moderate or severe OSA compared with ongoing medical management in continuous positive airway pressure (CPAP) failure.[2] Statistically significant improvement from baseline in the surgical group compared with ongoing medical management group was found in both apnea–hypopnea index (-27 vs. -10) (events/h) and ESS (−7 vs.−0.5). Secondary outcomes including other quality of life (snoring severity and sleep-specific and global quality of life) as well as apnea index, oxygen desaturation index, and time spent below 90% oxygen saturation all improved with surgery compared with control. At a mean of 3.5 years follow-up, outcomes were maintained.[3]

Overall long-term adverse events were minor; almost all patients in the surgical arm indicated they would recommend the surgery, and 69% of control patients subsequently underwent surgery with symptom and quality-of-life improvements. The accompanying graph indicates the improvement in almost all surgical patients in coprimary outcomes long term (**Fig. 1**).

SKUP3 Trial—2013

Browaldh and colleagues published SKUP3 in 2013 as a single-center prospective trial with two parallel arms of 32 patients in the intervention group (upfront UPPP) and 33 in the control group.[4] After surgery, AHI decreased by 60% (average baseline 53.3 events/h to 21.1 events/h) compared with 11% (average baseline 52.6 events/h to 46.8 events/h) in the control group. The difference between groups was statistically significant.

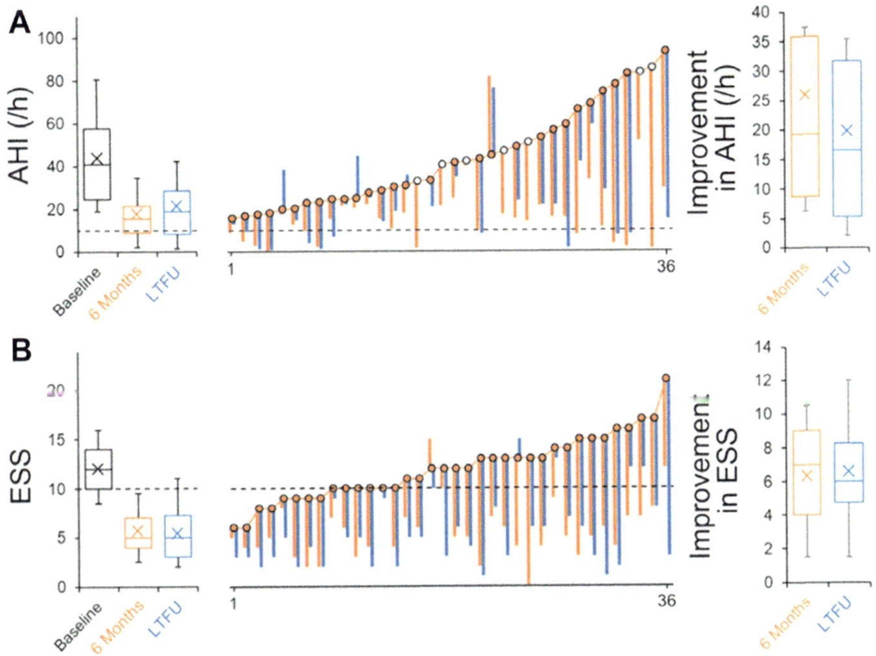

Fig. 1. AHI and ESS outcomes in SAMS LTFU study of the clinical effectiveness of modified uvulopalatopharyngoplasty and radiofrequency-in-saline tongue reduction for treatment of OSA. (*A*) AHI between baseline, 6 months and long term follow up (LTFU) following multi-level airway surgery. (*B*) ESS between baseline, 6 months and long term follow up (LTFU) following multi-level airway surgery (Alison J Pinczel et al., Sleep apnea multi-level surgery trial: long-term observational outcomes, Sleep, Volume 47, Issue 1, January 2024, zsad218, https://doi.org/10.1093/sleep/zsad218.)

Clinically important long-term follow-up results were achieved with surgery in the extended 8-year follow-up study.[5] In addition, two "spin off" studies identified both quality of life (QOL) *and* blood pressure (BP) improvements with pharyngeal surgery (QOL and BP studies).

Sommer Trial—2016

Two centers participated in a German randomized clinical trial in 2016 with 42 adult patients with OSA (AHI ≥15 events/h) unable to tolerate CPAP randomized to either tonsillectomy with their variant of UPPP or control.[6] The statistically significant and clinically relevant AHI reduction of 54% in the surgical group compared with 12% reduction in the control group was a key finding. Secondary outcomes (visual analog snoring scale and daytime somnolence) were also better with surgery compared with control.

CHAT Study—2013

In the CHAT study 226 five- to nine-year-olds with polysomnographically diagnosed mild to moderate OSA were randomly assigned to early adenotonsillectomy and 227 similar-aged children to watchful waiting.[7] At 7 months follow-up, CHAT reported 79% resolution of OSA in the early adenotonsillectomy group, along with statistically significant resolution of symptoms and parental assessment of outcome, compared with watchful waiting. Despite a lack of outcome in the curiously chosen NEPSY measure, surgery should remain the primary treatment modality based on polysomnogram and behavioral and other outcome measures.

Karolinska Adenotonsillectomy Study—2020

The Karolinska Adenotonsillectomy (KATE) RCT was designed to determine if early adenotonsillectomy is more effective than watchful waiting for treatment of mild to moderate OSA in children 2 to 4 years of age.[8] Children with moderate OSA (AHI >5 and < 10) experienced better AHI outcomes with early pharyngeal surgery than those in the watchful waiting group. Only minor differences between groups in mean obstructive AHI in favor of adenotonsillectomy were seen, but there were large improvements in quality of life after surgery.

PATS Study—2023

In a study of 458 children with mild sleep-disordered breathing, defined as habitual snoring without frequent obstructive events, adenotonsillectomy resulted in no statistically significant changes in executive function or attention but led to improved secondary outcomes including symptoms, behavior, and also BP.[9] A follow-up study found primary snoring and mild OSA difficult to distinguish in this cohort without polysomnography and on clinical indicators alone.[10]

Multiple Landmark Observational Studies and Systematic Review/Meta-Analyses

The past decade has also seen important studies using propensity score and cardinality matching,[11,12] supporting a role for pharyngeal surgery, others that suggest a role for earlier combinations of pharyngeal surgery,[13] and yet others measuring real-life outcomes such as modifying cardiovascular/diabetes risk with surgery.[14] A large volume of systematic reviews/meta-analyses have explored various types of pharyngeal surgery and found positive outcomes to support those operative interventions.[15–23]

ADVANCES IN SURGICAL TECHNIQUE

Most adult OSA pharyngeal surgeries involve soft tissue work to reposition the palate, and the last decade has seen published modified variants of UPPP that focus on antero-supero-lateral velopharyngeal port opening without resecting functional tissue.[4,24–26] Some investigators have even compared some of these newer techniques with variations of each other.[27] Anatomic understanding of the lateral palatal space has enhanced the theory behind these evolving palate surgeries.[28] Almost all of these techniques focus on a similar approach—mucosally preserving bilateral tonsillectomy, an approach to access the lateral palatal space or supra-tonsillar area, variations of releasing incisions, and supero-lateral advancement of portions of posterior pillar or palatopharyngeus with or without fixation as far up as pterygomandibular/pterygomaxillary raphe. Examples are shown in the following adaptations from the original publications (**Figs. 2–4**).

Transpalatal advancement in patients requiring more anterior repositioning or where a newer UPPP technique has been/is likely to be inadequate has more recently had its role solidified.[15] Despite its original description before the last decade, evolution of the procedure to include bony islands and finer piezo-drill pieces to reduce palatal fistula risk has occurred.[29]

Lower oropharyngeal surgeries have enjoyed a popularity spike in the last decade, particularly with newer technologies supporting access to reduction of such tissue as bulky lingual tonsils, both in pediatric and adult OSA.[30,31] Radiofrequency variants and

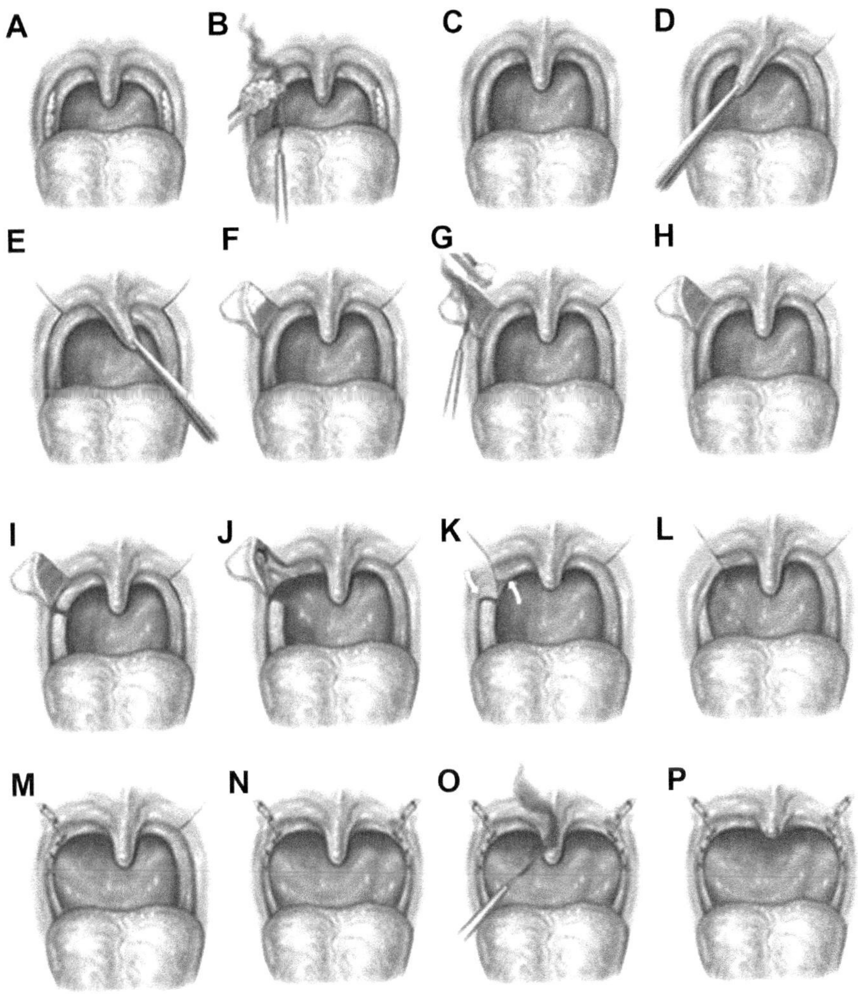

Fig. 2. Modified uvulopalatopharyngoplasty surgical technique (*A - P*). (MacKay, S. et al., (2013). Modified uvulopalatopharyngoplasty and coblation channeling of the tongue for obstructive sleep apnea: a Multi-Centre Australian trial. Journal of Clinical Sleep Medicine, 09(02), 117-124. https://doi.org/10.5664/jcsm.2402.)

coblation,[32,33] malleable suction diathermy, and similar implements permit greater access to these areas.

Reduction of macroglossia can be achieved by minimally invasive coblation channeling[24] or by a range of progressive mucosally preserving surgeries, such as midline glossectomy with or without lateral radiofrequency/coblation channeling or submucosal lingualplasty. Over the last decade these interventions have taken preference over traditional resective operations. Newer robotic techniques gained momentum (despite often incorporating posterior tongue mucosal sacrifice) but have tended to wane in popularity with the evolution of hypoglossal nerve stimulation options.[34]

Targeted epiglottic surgery has remained an option in multilevel surgery paradigms in the last 10 years, with some evolution in technology permitting ease of access (eg,

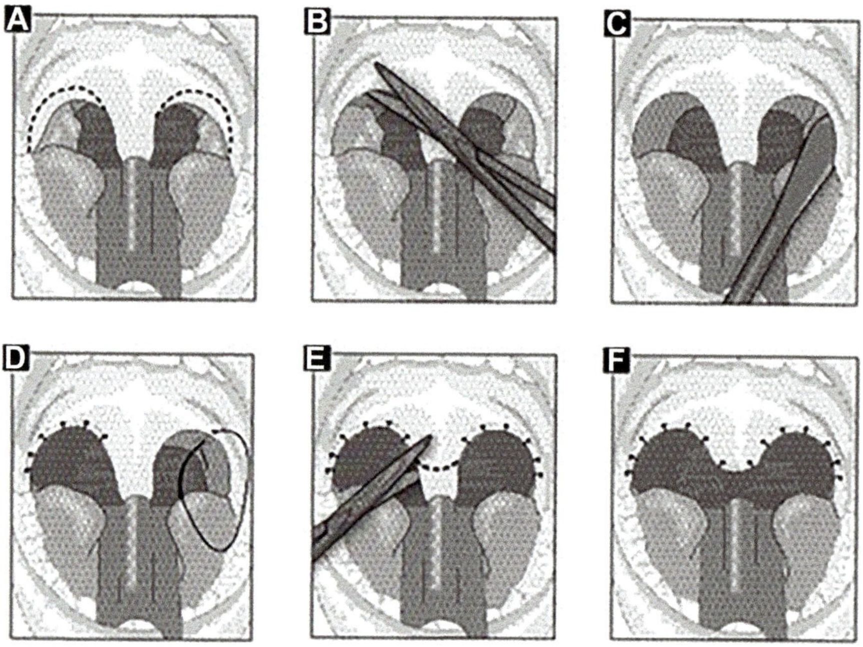

Fig. 3. Uvulopalatopharyngoplasty surgical technique (*A -F*). (*From* Browaldh N, Nerfeldt P, Lysdahl M, Bring J, Frieberg D. SKUP3 randomised controlled trial: polysomnographic results after uvulopalatopharyngoplasty in selected patients with obstructive sleep apnoea. Thorax. 2013;68(9):801-2.)

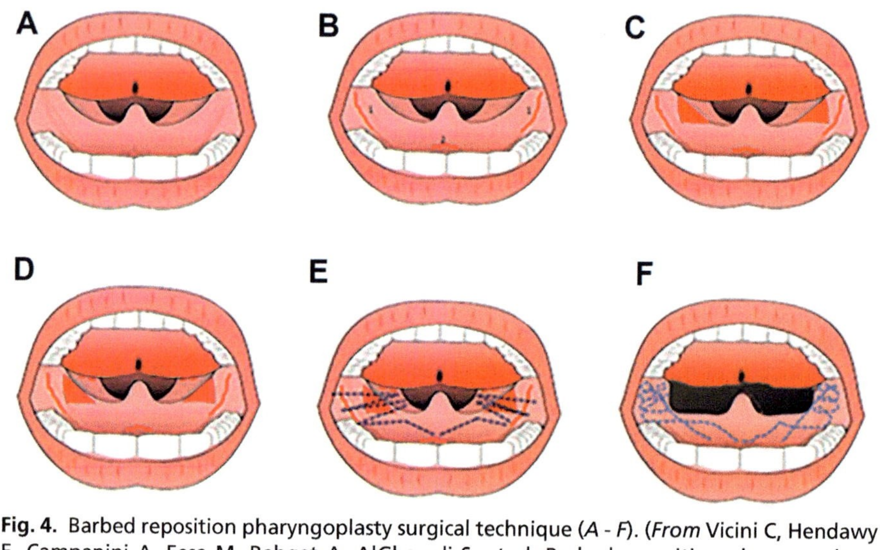

Fig. 4. Barbed reposition pharyngoplasty surgical technique (*A - F*). (*From* Vicini C, Hendawy E, Campanini A, Eesa M, Bahgat A, AlGhamdi S, et al. Barbed reposition pharyngoplasty (BRP) for OSAHS: a feasibility, safety, efficacy and teachability pilot study. "We are on the giant's shoulders". Eur Arch Otorhinolaryngol. 2015;272(10):3065-70.)

epiglottopexy with laparoscopic angled suture holders). Combined with recognition that in some cases CPAP may in fact exacerbate epiglottic collapse,[35,36] surgery might play an important role in either primary treatment or stabilization for repeat CPAP trial.

ADVANCES IN ASSESSMENT

Although the importance of history and static examination has been emphasized in various forums over the last decade, debate over how best to evaluate dynamic airway collapse (awake or asleep via drug-induced sleep endoscopy or via newer physiologic diagnostic tools) before contemporary pharyngeal surgery has taken center place. Well-executed multicenter studies designed to answer the disputes regarding drug-induced sleep endoscopy (DISE) have perhaps raised even more questions.[37] However, as a result of such research, there are likely dynamic phenotypes (eg, nontonsillar lateral pharyngeal wall collapse) that predict poorer pharyngeal surgical outcomes.

Comprehensive sleep history and examination paired with anatomical based algorithms have been developed, and allow appropriate selection of patients for pharyngeal surgery.[38]

In the pediatric population, equipoise regarding how to best manage residual sleep breathing disorders has led to National Institute of Health funding for a proposed anatomically DISE-directed study into multilevel pharyngeal surgery, soon to be underway.

ADVANCES IN COLLABORATION

Since 2013, collaborative groups have investigated the role of pharyngeal surgeries in mean disease alleviation,[11] evaluating surgical outcomes in various endophenotypes,[39] the importance of the pharyngeal surgeon in multidisciplinary care[40,41] and the ability pharyngeal surgery has to facilitate other treatments (convert to HGNS candidate). Evaluating means of marrying clinical assessment, anatomic findings, physiologic data, and endophenotypes into decision-making will drive further research.

Nationwide[2] and international collaborations[42] have established the role of pharyngeal surgeries in contemporary practice. These publications also advise upon newer, anatomically based algorithms in adult and pediatric OSA pharyngeal surgery; regarding adults, such paradigms seek to replace older staged protocols.[43]

FUTURE

In the era of established repositioning and minimally or nonresective pharyngeal surgeries, with robust supporting literature, the field is primed for recognition of the fact that such interventions can achieve mean disease alleviation and clinically important outcomes for adult patients and further salvage after adenotonsillectomy in the pediatric population.

CLINICS CARE POINTS

- Multi-level airway surgery demonstrates reduction in AHI, ESS (SAMS, SKUP3, Sommer) and long-term improvement which includes quality of life indices (SAMS LTFU).
- Pediatric OSA is treated primarily with adenotonsillectomy (CHAT, KATE, PATS).
- New measures of treatment outcome will likely enlighten our understanding of the role of pharyngeal surgery in OSA.

- Advances in OSA surgical technique is key.
- Robust patient and anatomical algorithms/selection are critical (within a multi-disciplinary group).

DISCLOSURE

S.G. Mackay is a consultant for CNXII, Invicta, Nyxoah and Inspire. Previous CI status on NHMRC, Australia, GPRWF, and IHMRI, Australia grants. J.D. Every has no disclosures.

REFERENCES

1. MacKay SG, Weaver EM. Surgery for adult obstructive sleep apnoea. Med J Aust 2013;199(7).
2. MacKay S, Carney AS, Catcheside PG, et al. Effect of Multilevel Upper Airway Surgery vs Medical Management on the Apnea-Hypopnea Index and Patient-Reported Daytime Sleepiness Among Patients With Moderate or Severe Obstructive Sleep Apnea: The SAMS Randomized Clinical Trial. JAMA 2020;324(12):1168–79.
3. Pinczel AJ, Woods CM, Catcheside PG, et al. Sleep Apnea Multi-level surgery trial: long term observational outcomes. Sleep 2023;47(1):zsad218.
4. Browaldh N, Nerfeldt P, Lysdahl M, et al. SKUP3 randomised controlled trial: polysomnographic results after uvulopalatopharyngoplasty in selected patients with obstructive sleep apnoea. Thorax 2013;68(9):801–2.
5. Sundman J, Browaldh N, Fehrm J, et al. Eight-Year Follow-up of Modified Uvulopalatopharyngoplasty in Patients With Obstructive Sleep Apnea. Laryngoscope 2021;131(1):E307–13.
6. Sommer UJ, Heiser C, Gahleitner C, et al. Tonsillectomy with Uvulopalatopharyngoplasty in Obstructive Sleep Apnea. Dtsch Arztebl Int 2016;113(1–02):1–8.
7. Marcus CL, Moore RH, Rosen CL, et al. A randomized trial of adenotonsillectomy for childhood sleep apnea. N Engl J Med 2013;368(25):2366–76.
8. Fehrm J, Nerfeldt P, Browaldh N, et al. Effectiveness of Adenotonsillectomy vs Watchful Waiting in Young Children With Mild to Moderate Obstructive Sleep Apnea: A Randomized Clinical Trial. JAMA Otolaryngol Head Neck Surg 2020;146(7):647–54.
9. Redline S, Cook K, Chervin RD, et al. Adenotonsillectomy for Snoring and Mild Sleep Apnea in Children: A Randomized Clinical Trial. JAMA 2023;330(21):2084–95.
10. Mitchell RB, Cook K, Garetz S, et al. Clinical Characteristics of Primary Snoring vs Mild Obstructive Sleep Apnea in Children: Analysis of the Pediatric Adenotonsillectomy for Snoring (PATS) Randomized Clinical Trial. JAMA Otolaryngology–Head & Neck Surgery 2023;150(2):99–106.
11. Every JD, Mackay SG, Sideris AW, et al. Mean disease alleviation between surgery and continuous positive airway pressure in matched adults with obstructive sleep apnea. Sleep 2023;46(9).
12. Ibrahim B, de Freitas Mendonca MI, Gombar S, et al. Association of Systemic Diseases With Surgical Treatment for Obstructive Sleep Apnea Compared With Continuous Positive Airway Pressure. JAMA Otolaryngol Head Neck Surg 2021;147(4):329–35.

13. Rotenberg BW, Theriault J, Gottesman S. Redefining the timing of surgery for obstructive sleep apnea in anatomically favorable patients. Laryngoscope 2014;124(Suppl 4):S1–9.
14. O'Connor-Reina C, Alcala LR, Ignacio JM, et al. Risk of diabetes in patients with sleep apnea: comparison of surgery versus CPAP in a long-term follow-up study. J Otolaryngol Head Neck Surg 2023;52(1):16.
15. Volner K, Dunn B, Chang ET, et al. Transpalatal advancement pharyngoplasty for obstructive sleep apnea: a systematic review and meta-analysis. Eur Arch Oto-Rhino-Laryngol 2017;274(3).
16. Camacho M, Li D, Kawai M, et al. Tonsillectomy for adult obstructive sleep apnea: A systematic review and meta-analysis. Laryngoscope 2016;126(9):2176–86.
17. Camacho M, Certal V, Brietzke SE, et al. Tracheostomy as treatment for adult obstructive sleep apnea: a systematic review and meta-analysis. Laryngoscope 2014;124(3):803–11.
18. Camacho M, Teixeira J, Abdullatif J, et al. Maxillomandibular advancement and tracheostomy for morbidly obese obstructive sleep apnea: a systematic review and meta-analysis. Otolaryngol Head Neck Surg 2015;152(4):619–30.
19. Song SA, Wei JM, Buttram J, et al. Hyoid surgery alone for obstructive sleep apnea: A systematic review and meta-analysis. Laryngoscope 2016;126(7):1702–8.
20. Camacho M, Zaghi S, Piccin O, et al. Expansion sphincter pharyngoplasty for obstructive sleep apnea: an update to the recent meta-analysis. Eur Arch Oto-Rhino-Laryngol 2016;273(9):2857–8.
21. Camacho M, Nesbitt NB, Lambert E, et al. Laser-Assisted Uvulopalatoplasty for Obstructive Sleep Apnea: A Systematic Review and Meta-Analysis. Sleep 2017;40(3).
22. Camacho M, Dunn B, Torre C, et al. Supraglottoplasty for laryngomalacia with obstructive sleep apnea: A systematic review and meta-analysis. Laryngoscope 2016;126(5):1246–55.
23. Llewellyn CM, Noller MW, Camacho M. Cautery-assisted palatal stiffening operation for obstructive sleep apnea: A systematic review and meta-analysis. World J Otorhinolaryngol Head Neck Surg 2019;5(1):49–56.
24. Mackay SG, Carney AS, Woods CM, et al. Modified Uvulopalatopharyngoplasty and Coblation channeling of the Tongue for Obstructive Sleep Apnea: A multi-centre Australian Trial. J Clin Sleep Med 2013;9(2).
25. Pang KP, Pang EB, Win MT, et al. Expansion sphincter pharyngoplasty for the treatment of OSA: a systemic review and meta-analysis. Eur Arch Oto-Rhino-Laryngol 2016;273(9):2329–33.
26. Vicini C, Hendawy E, Campanini A, et al. Barbed reposition pharyngoplasty (BRP) for OSAHS: a feasibility, safety, efficacy and teachability pilot study. "We are on the giant's shoulders". Eur Arch Oto-Rhino-Laryngol 2015;272(10):3065–70.
27. Neruntarat C, Khuancharee K, Saengthong P. Barbed reposition pharyngoplasty versus expansion sphincter pharyngoplasty: a meta-analysis. Laryngoscope 2020;131(6).
28. Woodson BT, Tadokoro KS, MacKay SG. Radiofrequency ablation of the lateral palatal space for snoring. World Journal of Otorhinolaryngology - Head and Neck Surgery 2017;3(2).
29. MacKay SG, Chan L. Surgical Approaches to Obstructive Sleep Apnea. Sleep Med Clin 2016;11(3):331–41.

30. Kang K, Koltai P, Lee C, et al. Lingual tonsillectomy for treatment of pediatric obstructive sleep apnea: a meta-analysis. JAMA Otolaryngol Head Neck Surg 2016;143(6).
31. Samutsakorn P, Hirunwiwatkul P, Chaitusaney B, et al. Lingual tonsillectomy with palatal surgery for the treatment of obstructive sleep apnea in adults: a systematic review and meta-analysis. Eur Arch Oto-Rhino-Laryngol 2018;275(4).
32. Li HY, Lee L, Kezirian E. Coblation endoscopic lingual lightning (CELL) for obstructive sleep apnea. Eur Arch Oto-Rhino-Laryngol 2015;273(1).
33. Pang KP, Rotenberg B, Woodson BT, editors. Advanced surgical techniques in snoring and obstructive sleep apnea. Plural Publishing; 2013.
34. Costantino A, Rinaldi V, Moffa A, et al. Hypoglossal nerve stimulation long-term clinical outcomes: a systematic review and meta-analysis. Sleep Breath 2019;24(2).
35. Dedhia RC, Rosen CA, Soose R. What is the role of the larynx in adult obstructive sleep apnea? Laryngoscope 2013;124(4).
36. Torre C, Camacho M, Liu SY, et al. Epiglottis collapse in adult obstructive sleep apnea: A systematic review. Laryngoscope 2016;126(2):515–23.
37. Green K, Kent D, D'Agostino MA, et al. Drug-Induced Sleep Endoscopy and Surgical Outcomes: A Multicenter Cohort Study. Laryngoscope 2018;129(3).
38. MacKay SG, Lewis R, McEvoy D, et al. Surgical management of obstructive sleep apnoea: A position statement of the Australasian Sleep Association. Respirology 2020;25(12):1292–308.
39. Joosten SA, Leong P, Landry SA, et al. Loop Gain Predicts the Response to Upper Airway Surgery in Patients With Obstructive Sleep Apnea. Sleep 2017;40(7).
40. MacKay S, Jefferson N, Jones A, et al. Benefit of a Contemporary Sleep Multidisciplinary Team (MDT): Patient and Clinician Evaluation. Journal of Sleep Disorders 2014;03(02).
41. Ouayoun MC, Chabolle F, De Vito A, et al. International consensus (ICON) on the ENT role in diagnosis of obstructive sleep apnea syndrome. Eur Ann Otorhinolaryngol Head Neck Dis 2018;135(1).
42. Chang JL, Goldberg AN, Alt JA, et al. International Consensus Statement on Obstructive Sleep Apnea. Int Forum Allergy Rhinol 2023;13(7):1061–482.
43. Riley RW, Powell NB, Guilleminault C. Obstructive sleep apnea syndrome: a surgical protocol for dynamic upper airway reconstruction. J Oral Maxillofac Surg 1993;51(7):742–7 [discussion 8-9].

9780443294068